The Business of Dentistry

Quintessentials of Dental Practice – 8
General Dentistry/Practice Management - 1

The Business of Dentistry

By
Raj Rattan
George Manolescue

Editor-in-Chief: Nairn H F Wilson
Editor General Dentistry/Practice Management: Raj Rattan

Quintessence Publishing Co. Ltd.

London, Berlin, Chicago, Copenhagen, Paris, Milan, Barcelona,
Istanbul, São Paulo, Tokyo, New Dehli, Moscow, Prague, Warsaw

British Library Cataloguing in Publication Data

Rattan, Raj
    The business of dentistry. - (The quintessentials of dental practice series. General dentistry/
    practice management; 1)
    1. Dentistry - Practice 2. Dental offices - Management
    I. Title II.Manolescue, George
    617.6'0068

    ISBN 1850970580

ISBN 1-85097-058-0

Foreword

For many practitioners, treating patients is relatively easy compared with the running of their practice as a successful business. With arrangements for the provision of oral healthcare undergoing dramatic changes, the need for dental practices to be efficient and effective businesses has probably never been greater. Patients must, however, come first, both ethically, to satisfy professional requirements of care, and as customers. As the authors of *The Business of Dentistry* point out on page 1, "look after your patients, then profits will follow".

For those practitioners who run the business aspects of their practice on a trial-and-error basis rather than according to sound principles of business management, this book – Volume 8 in the Quintessentials for General Dental Practitioners Series – will be a revelation. For practitioners who have and effectively apply good business acumen, this book will provide fresh impetus and encouragement to keep ahead of the field. It is a great achievement to prepare a book that motivates busy practitioners to stand back and rethink their approach to their patients, the running and development of their practice and the financial affairs of their business. *The Business of Dentistry* is such a book – a well-written, easy-to-read text in the succinct, essential style of the Quintessential Series, a book which can transform the reader's approach to the critically important interface between clinical dentistry and the management of a successful dental practice.

Nairn Wilson
Editor-in-Chief

Preface

Writing this book presented us with a challenge and a dilemma. The challenge was to adopt and adapt general business principles and make them relevant to dentistry. The dilemma was that we had more material than we could possibly hope to include given our editorial brief; it was a dilemma not of commission but of omission. The remaining titles in the General Dentistry and Practice Management volumes of the Quintessentials Series will examine some of the areas we have chosen to exclude from this particular text: risk management and dento-legal issues, quality assurance, teamwork, information technology and practice management.

Success in the world of business relies on effective and strong leadership – a theme which recurs in many modern texts on business management. According to Ridderstrale and Nordstrom's bestselling book, Funky Business, "leadership and management are more important than ever before" and are the "keys to competitive advantage". Their perspective is people-centred – "the most critical resource wears shoes and walks out of the door around five o'clock every day".

This book also draws its inspiration from the Chinese concept of Guanxi. "Guan" means "close together" and "Xi" means "relationship". Guanxi, then, is essentially about relationship management –widely recognised to be a key determinant of business performance. It is a prime example of one-to-one marketing and of customer relationship management (CRM). CRM has been defined as "the implementation of business strategies that identify and manage customers to derive maximum long-term value from that relationship", and it requires a "customer-centric business philosophy that is often a change from the traditional product-oriented nature of many businesses". Don't let the jargon mislead you – the principles are as old as civilisation itself.

Above all, we must recognise the most valuable aspect of the dental profession – that of being allowed to treat patients. The business of dentistry will reap rewards for those who recognise this for the privilege that it is and whose business is nourished by high ethical standards. Contrary to popular belief – and despite the spate of recent high-profile failures in the corporate world – success in business does not require abandoning high ethical standards. According to The Institute of Business Ethics, "a business that doesn't invest in building trust will, over time, be rejected by the markets, by investors, by its customers and above all by its own people – its employees". We must remember that ethical considerations are inseparable from, and inextricably linked to, the business of dentistry.

Raj Rattan

Acknowledgements

It has been privilege to work with my colleagues on the editorial board of this series – their individual and collective enthusiasm has been an inspiration throughout, as has that of the team at Quintessence Publishing.

I am grateful to Dental Design and Planning Consultants Ltd. in London who provided the colour photographs of their interior design work for inclusion in this book.

Contents

Chapter 1
What Business Are We In?

The purpose of any business is to generate profit. The view that health care and profit generation are somehow mutually exclusive and require the providers of healthcare to abandon their commitment to clinical quality and to uphold the highest professional ethics is one myth which should be dismissed from the outset.

The business of dentistry is about providing high-quality clinical care in a high-quality environment. The challenge in the business of dentistry is to provide it profitably and in a way that makes patients appreciate and value the treatment they receive. To meet this challenge we must apply the principles of commerce. We must have an understanding of the meaning and purpose of marketing, knowledge of human psychology and an appreciation that the title of "patient" confers a special status on any member of the public whose behaviour will be that of a dental "consumer" or "client".

Customer or Patient?

There is no need to deliberate as to whether we should call our patients "customers", "consumers" or "clients" because they are all three. What makes them patients is the ethical bond and duty of care that attaches them to the healthcare profession. We will use all these terms in this text to reflect the origins of the principles that are under discussion. We must remember that in any business high levels of profitability and growth are primarily stimulated, driven and sustained by customer loyalty. The business of dentistry is no exception.

Patient Care and Profit

In this book we have chosen to take the view that if you look after your patients, then the profits will follow. In so doing we must understand the meaning of "looking after". But we must remember that there is more to looking after people than looking after their teeth, and when we create the environment in which we want to "look after" them, then we must be sure that that environment is built on a sound business principles with profit gen-

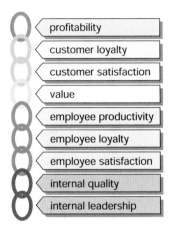

Fig 1-1 The service profit chain.

eration in mind. No profit means no practice and we lose the opportunity of looking after people.

The Service Profit Chain

In 1994, Heskett developed the concept of the "service profit chain" (Fig 1-1). Its core principles demonstrate perfectly the key linkages that are the business of dentistry. The service profit chain, developed from analyses of successful service organisations, helped to establish the relationships between profitability, customer loyalty, employee satisfaction and productivity. Further exploration of these relationships led to the publication in 1997 of Heskett, Sasser and Schlesinger's book *The Service Profit Chain: How Leading Companies Link Profit and Growth to Loyalty, Satisfaction, and Value*. We can adapt its customer-orientation slant and make it relevant to the business of dentistry (Fig 1-2).

This approach demonstrates that there are strong links between:
profit and patient loyalty
employee loyalty and patient loyalty
employee satisfaction and patient satisfaction.

Mission Statement

One way to communicate and share your vision is to prepare a mission statement. Mission statements have become a part of business culture and many

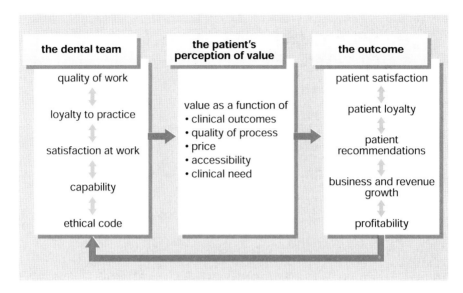

Fig 1-2 The service profit link.

dentists have adopted this practice. Your mission statement should be able to tell your practice story in less than thirty seconds. Here are ten tips to help you create an effective mission statement.

1. An effective mission statement should state who you are, what you do, and what you stand for.
2. Remember your mission statement is not a slogan or an advert.
3. An effective mission statement is best developed with input from all the team. Even if certain members think it is silly or have no ideas (both are common), they will buy into the concept more if their opinion is solicited.
4. Take time to create your mission statement. Put it away and look at it again a week later and refine it.
5. Look at other mission statements to get some ideas. (Do not copy your statement: it has to be about *you*.)
6. Keep the statement simple and honest. Avoid humour and grandiloquence. (Aim for between one and four sentences.)
7. Avoid saying how great you are or what great quality and what great service your practice provides. (Using such clichés makes you indistinguishable from the rest. Have you ever seen any business say otherwise?)

3

8. You must believe in your statement. If you do not believe it, then it is a lie and your patients will know it is a lie.
9. Use your mission statement to supplement your marketing communications.
10. Make certain everyone in the practice gets a copy of the statement. Use your mission statement in your staff manual and at practice meetings, and post it in the practice.

Some examples of phrases used by dental bodies corporate in their mission statements are shown in Table 1-1.

Table 1-1. **Approach to customer care (from Newsome, PRH. Dental bodies corporate and their approach to customer care. BDJ 2002;192:572-575)**

Treatment-related	"quality dental care"; "highest quality of care through sophisticated treatment modalities".
Patient-centred	"putting patients first"; "dental care with you in mind"; "emphasis on excellent patient careaffordable"
Environmental (practice and staff)	"supportive environment"; "friendly and relaxed atmosphere"; "state-of-the-art practices"; "efficient and highly focussed team"

The Nuts and Bolts of the Business of Dentistry

The nuts and bolts of the business of dentistry are no different from those of any other business. To succeed, you must have:
- leadership
- vision
- effective teamwork
- business acumen
- an understanding of services and products
- customer focus.

Leadership and Vision

Dr John C. Maxwell, author of *The 21 Irrefutable Laws of Leadership*, notes, "everything rises or falls on leadership". He describes a good leader as someone who "knows the way, goes the way and shows the way" and observed that a good leader takes a little more than his share of the blame and a little less than his share of the credit. In your practice, good leadership is about setting direction – sometimes a change of direction. It is about clarifying your vision, helping your team to share that vision and motivating them to want to achieve it. Vision is about the future. It is where we will all spend the rest of our life.

As a leader in your business, you should have the ability to:
- Challenge processes. Find a process that you believe needs to be improved the most and act on it.
- Share your vision with the team.
- Enable and empower your team to act.
- Model the way. A "boss" simply tells others what to do; a "leader" demonstrates it can be done.
- Inspire. Share success with your team. Keep the pain to yourself.

In ten short chapters on "developing the leader within you", Maxwell summarises what leadership is all about. He concludes that:
- The definition of leadership is *influence*.
- The key to leadership is about *setting priorities*.
- The most important ingredient of leadership is *integrity*.
- The ultimate test of leadership lies in *creating positive change*.
- The quickest way to gain leadership is to *problem solve*.
- The extra plus in leadership is *attitude*.
- Your most appreciable asset is your *people*.
- The indispensable quality of leadership is *vision*.
- The price tag of leadership is *self-discipline*.
- The most important lesson of leadership is to commit to *staff development*.

History reveals many inspired visions, and few are as remarkable as that of John F Kennedy when on 25 May 1961 during a joint session of Congress he shared his vision for the United States: "I believe that this nation should commit itself to achieving the goal, before this decade is out, of landing a man on the moon and returning him safely to the Earth." The team at NASA realised that goal (although John F Kennedy did not live to see his vision become reality).

There are essentially three styles of leadership. The styles and their characteristics are summarised in Table 1-2. Another useful model is to look at the

Table 1-2. **Three styles of leadership**

Autocratic	Authoritarian. Decisions are made without consultation - a very dictatorial approach to decision-making. Can make others in the team feel isolated and alienated.
Democratic	A participative approach. Decisions are made jointly and team involvement is encouraged. The team is made to feel important and has ownership of decisions and outcomes.
Laissez-faire	Sometimes known as the "permissive" style of leadership - there is abdication of responsibility and lack of control. The business has no real direction.

preferred focus of the leader: are you people-focused or output-focused? This relationship can be explored in a model developed by Robert Blake and Jane Mouton in 1964 known as the managerial grid (Fig 1-3). In this model, the 2-2 style shows little concern for people or output and may reflect a permissive approach to practice management. The 3-9 style is people-focused, but if there is insufficient focus on output, then the financial status of the practice may be vulnerable. This position is difficult to sustain, particularly if practice costs are not being met. The 9-9 approach is clearly a winning strategy – and reflects a "win-win" approach to leadership thinking.

Kurt Lewin is known for carrying out some pioneering research into the effectiveness of leadership. Although the research was carried out in the 1930s, many of his findings form the basis of modern business practice. Lewin

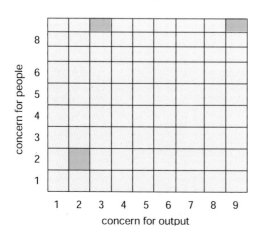

Fig 1-3 The managerial grid.

observed how groups performed when led by individuals who adopted the different styles of leadership: "laissez faire", "autocratic" or "democratic". A laissez-faire style produced the least work that was also of the poorest quality. In the group that had been exposed to the autocratic leader, some group members became submissive and other showed hostility towards the leader. Interestingly, the group members did not complain during the exercise but expressed their concerns in the debriefing interviews afterwards. It is a common observation in organisations that in the absence of an overly autocratic leader, employees take the opportunity to "have a go at the Boss". The members of the democratic group were more interested in their work and continued to work well when their leader left the room – in contrast to the other two groups. In reality, a combination of styles works best depending on the situation. The idea of benign autocracy is appealing to those who wish to retain control over goals, but the democratic style may prevail during discussions and decision-making.

Effective Teamwork

The business of dentistry is totally dependent on the effectiveness of your team. The team must trust and respect one another and they must respect and trust you. To help build this relationship, you should
• Be totally professional in your attitude.
• Accept responsibility.
• Demonstrate competence, honesty, integrity and candour.
• Know your strengths and weaknesses.
• Understand the human side of the business – this business is about people.
• Update your knowledge of clinical dentistry.
• Understanding the principles of business management.
• Provide direction by goal setting, problem solving and decision-making.
• Implement new initiatives.
• Respect and support your team.

There is research evidence to show that trust and confidence in leadership are the two most reliable predictors of employee satisfaction in any organisation.

Business Acumen

Business acumen is an essential ingredient for success in the business of dentistry. It is about having an understanding of how a business operates, why

businesses succeed and why they fail. It is also about:
- Seeking to create opportunities that add value to the business.
- Conducting business in a professional way.
- Making strategic and operational decisions by evaluating and managing risk based on business principles.
- Exercising sound judgement.
- Honesty and integrity.
- Adhering closely to your principles.
- Having proper regard for professional ethics.

Understanding Products and Services

The products of dentistry are the crowns, the individual restorations, the fixed and removable prostheses, the root canal treatments and so on. Patients are rarely interested in the features and advantages of these products (which are of great importance to the dentist), they are more interested in the benefits. The way these are delivered accounts for the service element of the business.

When giving choice of products to patients, the focus of our communications should relate to the benefits for the patient as derived from an evidence-based perspective, not from a commercial standpoint. In other words, we are dealing with a *patient* here and not a *customer,* although the patient may share many of the characteristics of a customer in other ways. Choice concerning products can be modelled on a commercial view. In *Strategic Marketing for Nonprofit Organizations* Kotler and Andreasen (1991) put products into three categories (Fig 1-4):
- the core product
- the tangible product
- the augmented product.

Core products meet underlying need. They provide the essentials and little more. A patient who loses an amalgam restoration can have it replaced with a similar restoration. The cavity is restored, the tooth is functional and a core product has satisfied the need. Tangible products can be looked upon as enhanced core products. In the example quoted, it might be a composite restoration if such a restoration was an appropriate option. Augmented products provide further enhancements – a ceramic material, for example. They may involve additional guarantees and include additional service elements. One example might be a 24-hour turnaround time for constructing a crown for a patient. This concept of the product is explored further in Chapter 5.

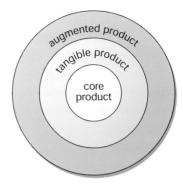

Fig 1-4 Product analysis.

Historically, the business of dentistry has focused on product provision when treatment needs and demand determined the trend. Dental students are taught in a product-centred way and item-of-service payment systems reward a product-centred approach. Very few businesses (if any at all) can be classified as solely service or product based. There are some businesses where service components are greater or less than those of others. Today, an educated public places increasing emphasis on the service elements of delivery. Kotler and Armstrong define a service as " an activity or benefit that one party can offer to another that is essentially intangible and does not result in ownership of anything. Its production may or may not be tied to a physical product." It is described as intangible because service cannot be assessed in the physical sense. Unlike a product, it has no appearance, smell, taste, shape or physical form, but it is easily recognised. Professor Robert Dailey of Edinburgh Business School makes the observation that "differentiating service is easier and faster than changing the physical features of products".

According to the work of Parasuraman, Zeithaml and Berry, there are five dimensions to a quality service. These are summarised in Table 1-3.

Consumer research suggests that:
- 30% of consumers see *good service* as doing what you say you will do.
- 25% mention doing it quickly – faster than they expect.
- 20% emphasise repeated experience of good service.
- 8% mention pleasant and friendly manners.

It would not be unreasonable to suggest that patients would have a similar perspective. It is worth remembering that patients judge quality on the basis

Table 1-3. Five dimensions of a quality service (from Parasuraman, Berry, Zeithaml, SERVQUAL: A multiple-item scale for measuring customer perceptions of service quality)

Dimensions of Quality	What Does This Mean in Practice?
Dependability	*Did you do what you promised?* With treatment planning, much of what the patient agrees to relies on what the dentist has said or indicated. The patient "buys into" the care on promise but will measure the outcome on delivery.
Responsiveness	*Was the service provided in a timely manner?* This means at a time convenient to the patient and within a time frame, which suited the patient's wishes. Did you always run late? Was the work from the laboratory on time and not delayed?
Authority	*Did you elicit a feeling of confidence in the patient?* Were you organised with the treatment? Did it look as though you knew what you were doing? Did you have the answers to the patient's questions?
Empathy	*Were you able to see the situation from the patient's point of view?* Did you understand how they felt about the situation and what was important to them during their treatment? Were you able to share in their concerns and worries?
Tangible evidence	*Is there evidence to show that you performed?* What is the outcome of the treatment? Is the patient able to easily visualise or sense the benefits of treatment?

of what is delivered and not on what was promised. In other words, you cannot rely on your mission statement for support if your practice fails to deliver what was promised. This is discussed more fully in Chapter 3.

Based on work carried out in competitive service industries, we can draw a number of conclusions that apply in the business of dentistry. These are:
- The quality of the service is relative and not absolute.
- The quality of the service is determined by the patient and not by the dentist or other team members.
- The perception of quality will differ from one patient to another depending on their baseline expectation.
- Improvements in service quality will only be perceived if a patient's expectations are at least met (or, preferably, exceeded). This may mean managing the expectation in the first place if it is unrealistic.

We can also draw from the work of Tom Peters. His book *Liberation Management* was published in 1992 and its guiding tenets for professional service organisations continue to apply. Amongst these are the following seven characteristics:

1. *"Adhocracy" is the norm.* The message is to be fluid and change with the market whilst still maintaining core values. In the business of dentistry the ethical value should prevail irrespective of market conditions.
2. *Follow personal interests.* Peters observes that the professional environment is organised according to the personal interests of key players. The same is true in dentistry where the practice becomes an extension of the personality of the principals.
3. *Create an "all–report–to–all" structure to avoid hierarchy.* This does not mean abandon leadership, but is an observation that the traditional line management reporting structure does not appear to apply to professional businesses. "Today's boss is tomorrow's subordinate and vice versa."
4. *Specialisation is critical.* This is concerned with professional expertise in a niche market. The dental profession already operates in a niche market and the recent introduction of Specialist Lists creates a micro-niche-market segment within the existing structure. It takes Peters' observation one stage further.
5. *Relationship management is essential*. This is concerned with nurturing relationships with major clients (our patients).
6. *The client is king.* Every patient in your practice is special and important and the aim is to foster a symbiotic relationship. Peters notes that all first-rank professional service firms are organised around the customer, just as

in dentistry many practices gear their opening hours to suit the preferences of patients. At one time, extended opening hours and Sunday clinics were unheard of but are now commonplace in many areas.

7. ***Methodology is philosophy***. Professional service organisations depend on core technologies that help them to problem solve, and we should not forget that outdated technologies hinder progress. Where is your practice positioned in relation to this particular guiding tenet?

Customer Focus

Good service is not a substitute for poor product quality. In his book *Customers for Life* Carl Sewell makes the observation that "Being nice to people is just 20% of providing good customer service. All the smiles in the world are not going to help you if your product or service is not what the customer wants". Creating a patient-centred practice is the key to business success. It is discussed more fully in Chapter 3.

Business Planning

Business planning relies on understanding some fundamental concepts and having access to a range of resources that are essential for your success. Of the many, we have selected three that we believe are essential in the business of dentistry:

- The Sigmoid curve
- The Gantt chart
- Pareto's principle.

The Sigmoid curve

There are many business patterns relevant to the business of dentistry, and none is more relevant than the concept behind the Sigmoid curve, shown in Fig 1-5. The Sigmoid curve is the S-shaped curve that has intrigued people throughout history.

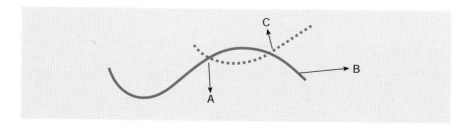

Fig 1-5 The Sigmoid curve.

> "The curve sums up the story and time line of life itself;
> we start slowly, we experiment and falter, we then grow
> rapidly, then wax, and wane. It describes the rise and fall
> of empires, dynasties, companies, and individuals."
> (Charles Handy, *The Age of Paradox*)

It has been suggested that competitive organisations perpetuate growth by creating an organisation within an organisation on a cyclical basis. The Sigmoid curve is flat or shows a downturn at the inception of a company, curves upward as the organisation experiences growth, begins to plateau as the business matures and then turns south as the business starts to decline. To maintain growth and profitability, the downturn should be prevented and, according to Handy, "the right place to start that second curve (shown by the dotted line) is at point A. At this point, there is the time, as well as the resources and the energy, to get the new curve through its initial explorations and floundering before the first curve begins to dip downwards". Ideally, point C – the growth phase of the second curve – should coincide with some point in the plateau of the first curve.

The Gantt chart
Your practice will undergo phases of development and refurbishment. How you handle and co-ordinate these are important aspects of the business of dentistry. Poorly planned and executed surgery installation can cause unnecessary delays in the schedule, and, in the business of dentistry, time is money. The Gantt chart is a useful project-planning tool. It can be used to represent the timing of tasks required to complete a project. Essentially a bar chart, it is a useful aide-mémoire of where the project stands, but is only in fact a static representation of a dynamic situation. An example of a completed project relating to a surgery installation is shown in Fig 1-6.

Gantt charts are simple to understand and easy to construct and are used by most project managers for all but the most complex projects. Each task takes up one row in the chart. Dates run along the top in increments of days, weeks or months, depending on the total length of the project. The expected time for each task is represented by a horizontal bar whose left end marks the expected beginning of the task and whose right end marks the expected completion date. Tasks may run sequentially, in parallel or overlapping. As the

programme of works: refurbisment of surgery 3

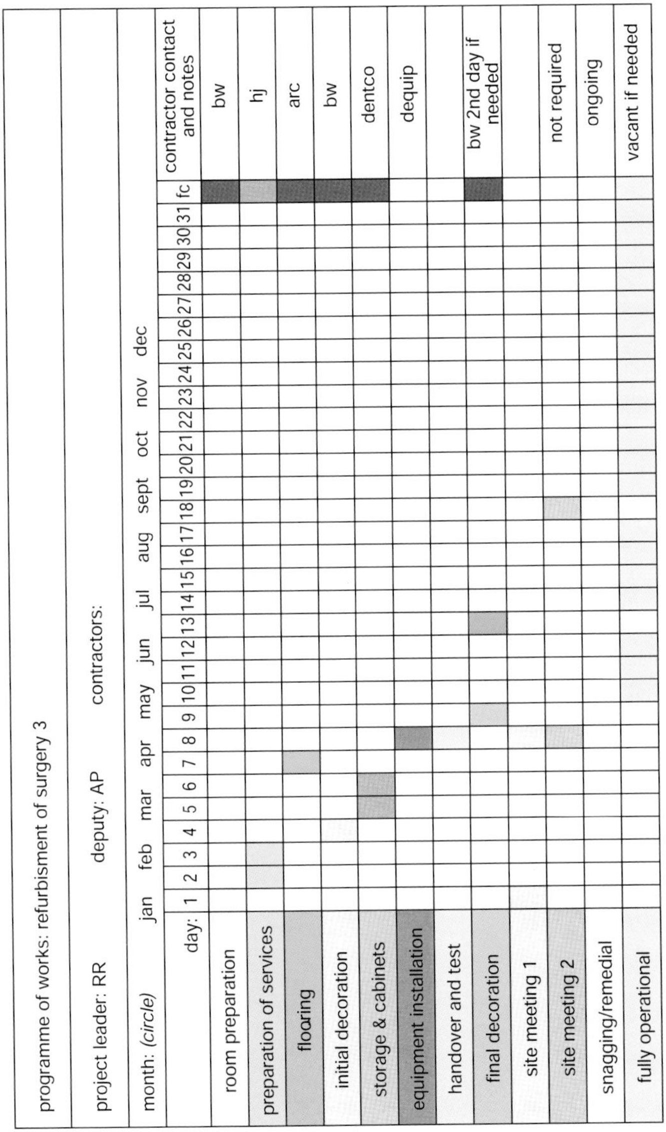

project leader: RR   deputy: AP   contractors:

month: (circle)   jan feb mar apr may jun jul aug sept oct nov dec

day:	1 2 3 4 5 6 7 8 9 10 11 12 13 14 15 16 17 18 19 20 21 22 23 24 25 26 27 28 29 30 31	fc	contractor contact and notes
room preparation			bw
preparation of services			hj
flooring			arc
initial decoration			bw
storage & cabinets			dentco
equipment installation			dequip
handover and test			
final decoration			bw 2nd day if needed
site meeting 1			not required
site meeting 2			
snagging/remedial			ongoing
fully operational			vacant if needed

Fig 1-6 The Gantt chart.

project progresses, the chart is updated by filling in the bars to a length proportional to the fraction of work that has been accomplished. This way one can get a quick reading of project progress by drawing a vertical line through the chart at the current date. Completed tasks lie to the left of the line and are completely filled in. Current tasks will lie across the line and are behind schedule if their filled-in section is to the left of the line or ahead of schedule if the filled-in section stops to the right of the line. Future tasks lie completely to the right of the line.

Pareto's principle

Vilfredo Pareto was an Italian economist and sociologist working at the end of the nineteenth century. He formulated something he called "the law of the unequal distribution of results" based on his observation that approximately 80% of the wealth in Italy was distributed amongst 20% of the population. It is more commonly known as the 80/20 rule. All the 80/20 rule says is that 20% of your effort will give you 80% of the results. The trick is finding that 20%, and once you have found it, paying attention to it.

Pareto's observation failed to receive the recognition it deserved until George Zipf, a Harvard professor of philosophy, came up with his "principle of least effort". Predictably, his concept struck a cord in society. Zipf went on to reframe Pareto's observation and expressed the concept in terms of productivity where 20-30% of a resource (human or otherwise) accounted for 70-80% of the activity related to that resource (see Fig 1-7).

The exact ratio is not particularly significant – it could be 30/70 – what is important is to recognise the leverage that holds true in many situations. For example:
- In commercial terms, 20% of a company's products may account for 80%

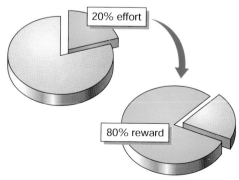

Fig 1-7 The 80/20 rule.

of its profits.
- In computer software, 20% of the features are used 80% of the time.
- In a restaurant, 80% of the meals come from 20% of the menu.

If 20% of a person's effort generates 80% of the results then the corollary is that 20% of the results we achieve take up some 80% of our effort. The challenge in the business of dentistry is to identify the vital 20% from the trivial 80%.

Consider these ten observations as a challenge of your effective leadership:
- 80% of the key decisions in meetings arise from only 20% of the meeting time.
- 80% of your practice management time is spent on 20% of tasks.
- 80% of complaints are about the same 20% of services.
- 20% of your advertising or marketing initiatives will produce 80% of your results.
- 80% of staff problems arise from 20% of your team members.
- 80% of absences arise from the same 20% of the team.
- 80% of your success comes from 20% of your efforts.
- 80% of clinical failures will be on 20% of your patients.
- 80% of your annual equipment repair bill will be generated by 20% of your equipment.
- 20% of the business of dentistry will occupy 80% of your time.

The value of this observation to any individual or organisation determined to achieve more is to note that if you could double your top 20% of activities you could work a two-day week and achieve 60% more.

The Planning Hierarchy

The different disciplines discussed in this chapter interrelate in what can be described as a planning hierarchy with a "top-down" approach to business planning (see Fig 1-8). Ask yourself the following sets of questions to bring these elements together.
- Where do you want to be in five years' time? Consider clinical trends, business trends but also the business aspects of your practice. How many surgeries? What blend of skill mix do you want in the team?
- How realistic and achievable is the vision?

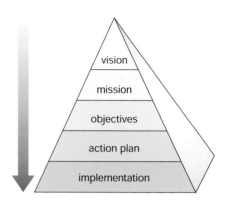

1-8 A top-down approach to business planning.

- What do you need to do to make the vision a reality? How does that fit in with your vision for your personal life and your family?

Further Reading

Blake RR, Mouton JS. The Managerial Grid. Houston, TX: Gulf Publishing Company, 1964.

Handy C. The Age of Paradox. Cambridge, MA: Harvard Business School Press, 1994.

Heskett JL, Sasser WE, Schlesinger LA. Service Profit Chain: How Leading Companies Link Profit and Growth to Loyalty, Satisfaction, and Value. New York: The Free Press, 1997.

Heskett JL. Putting the service profit chain to work. Harvard Bus Rev 1994;Mar.-Apr.:164-174.

Kotler P, Andreasen A. Strategic Marketing for Nonprofit Organizations. 4th Ed. Englewood Cliffs, NJ: Prentice-Hall, 1991.

Kouzes J, Posner, B. The Leadership Challenge: How to Get Extraordinary Things Done in Organizations. San Francisco: Jossey-Bass Inc., 1987.

Lewin K, Lippitt R, White RK. Patterns of aggressive behavior in experimentally created social climates. J Social Psychol 1939;10:271-279.

Maxwell JC. The 21 Irrefutable Laws of Leadership. Nashville, TN: Thomas Nelson, 1998.

Parasuraman A, Berry LL, Zeithaml, VA. SERVQUAL: A multiple-item scale for measuring customer perceptions of service quality. J Retail 1988;64:12-40.

Parasuraman A, Zeithaml VA, Berry LL. A conceptual model of service quality and its implications for future research. J Market 1985;49:41-50.
Peters T. Liberation Management. London: Pan, 1992.

Sewell C. Customers for Life. New York: Doubleday Currency, 1990.

Zipf GK. Human Behavior and the Principle of Least Effort: An Introduction to Human Ecology. New York: Hafner, 1965.

Chapter 2
Success Factors

Success in business is rarely accidental or incidental. It should be a planned outcome. In dentistry, it is a function of your reputation and your business acumen; combine the two and you will experience synergy at work. Your professional reputation will play a big part in the success of your business and the best way to gain a good reputation, according to Socrates, is "to endeavour to be what you desire to appear".

What is Success?

Howard Whitman wrote, "Success is no straitjacket. It is no mould into which all must be poured. It is no rigid stamp. It is as individual as our fingerprints or the look in our eyes." In other words, success should be about what you want to achieve in your chosen profession. There is no magic formula, but there is a recipe because success for most dentists is a blend of the following:
* professional status
* postgraduate qualifications
* financial security
* personal life-style
* family matters
* freedom of choice.

This list is not intended to be exhaustive or indeed given in order of preference. It represents a number of destinations, all of which are part of a professional and personal journey.

Metrics are important – we all need to know where we are, where we are going and how long it will take to get there. Prioritise your destinations and then plan the route. Stay focused, because, as someone once said, the road to success is lined with many tempting parking spaces.

Critical Success Factors

Critical success factors are those things that an organisation must be successful in achieving in order to grow, become viable and flourish in the commercial marketplace. In other words, they are the factors most responsible for your practice's success. The future prosperity of your practice will depend on them. Business failure is usually the result of one (or, frequently, a combination) of the following:

- Lack of planning.
- Setting unrealistic expectations.
- Not understanding the customer. (Changes in your patients' preferences and your competitors' products and services can leave you behind the curve.)
- Getting wedded to an idea and sticking with it for too long. (Do not marry a single idea. Remember that ideas are the currency of entrepreneurs. Play with many ideas and see which ones produce positive outcomes.)
- No Marketing Plan. (A marketing plan creates the kind of attention you need to get in front of the right types of people, companies, etc.)
- Ignoring Employees. (Expenditure on the team is an investment and not an unnecessary expense. Motivating, coaching and managing your staff are probably the toughest challenges in any business. Lack of morale and motivation can rapidly erode profits.)
- Confusing likelihood with reality. (The successful entrepreneur lives in a world of likelihood but remember that expenditure takes place in the world of reality.)
- Not moving with the times. (Where your business is today is down to what you did yesterday. Times change, so remember that yesterday's success was based on yesterday's strategy and that is no guarantee that tomorrow will be the same.)
- Focusing on new customers and ignoring your existing ones.
- Fear of change.

In general terms, business success relies on focusing on the four Cs:
- controls and measurement
- cost analysis
- cash management
- customer care.

The four Cs are also central to this book.

When patients return to seek their care and treatment at your practice, they bring you business. They do so for a number of reasons, but there are usually only a few critical ones. Without these, they would not come to you. There may be other reasons, but they may not make a lot of difference. When dentists are asked why patients continue to come to them the reasons most often cited are:

- The patients are given good value.
- The dentists are reliable.
- The quality of dentistry is good.
- There is a high level of customer care.

Now take a look at any practice information leaflet or read any advertisement in a business directory and you find that most practices (if not all) list the above as key features of their practice. Patients hear and read the same things from everyone. So what makes *your* practice special?

Identify your critical success factors by following the sequence shown in Table 2-1. Factors common to all practices are shown in Table 2-2. Every dentist has one critical success factor unique to their practising environment and one that no one else can ever copy. That factor is *you*.

The success of your business depends initially on the financial framework that has been put in place to support it (Fig 2-1), but then on your **m**otivation, your **a**bility and your **p**ersonal qualities – the MAP for your unique journey.

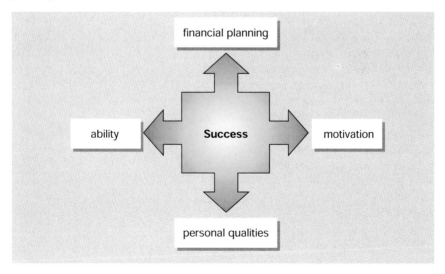

Fig 2-1 Financial framework of your business.

Table 2-1. **Identifying your critical success factors**

Step 1 Ask your patients	You want to concentrate on areas that your patients find critical and which make them choose you. The best way to do this is to ask them! They will give you feedback and tell you what they would like to see. Once you have discussed your practice with some of your most loyal and valued patients, you will notice a pattern - groups of patients will value the same things.
Step 2 Measure	Your next step is to establish a measurement scale for each critical factor. Everything is measurable, you just need the right system. Some of these measures will be quantitative and some qualitative. Gross fee income is an easy one – measuring revenue measured against realistic targets and budgets for expenditure. The number of new patient inquiries is also something that is easy to measure.
Step 3 Set the baseline be	Once you've established a measurement structure for a factor, the next step is setting a baseline. Each factor should set against a scale ranging from 1 to 10. Subjectively this can translate into poor performing (1), poor (2-3), mediocre (4-5), good (6-7), excellent (8-9), and exemplary (10). You decide on the scoring and we must accept that this is a subjective process.
Step 4 Set new goals	You should now create a "gap" between where you are - your baseline - and your target for that factor. If you want to control expenditure in a certain area of your practice, your current position may be 5 but you want to aim at 8. The same approach can apply foe developing your clinical skills and staff training initiatives. Your goals will have an impact on how you allocate your resources and energy. To help you prioritise which areas you want to focus on, look at return on investment, required resources, scheduling conflicts, time to impact, total cost, and likelihood of success versus risk of failure.

Step 5	You now have a baseline and a target for each factor and
Close the gap	your challenge is to close it. Ask the question: What will close the gap between our current level of this factor and our desired level? What actions are required to raise the subjective measurement to meet the target?

Table 2-2. Critical success factors common to all practices

1. Positive attitude toward work
2. Proficiency in the clinical dentistry
3. Good communication skills (verbal, non-verbal and written)
4. Interpersonal skills
5. Self-confidence
6. Critical thinking and problem solving skills
7. Flexibility
8. Self-motivation
9. Leadership
10. Teamwork

Ability

Ability is made up of knowledge skills and attitude, and in the business of dentistry attitude is much more important than aptitude. The first and most important thing you need to acquire in order to succeed in the business of dentistry is knowledge. According to research conducted by Dun and Bradstreet, one of the world's leading providers of business information, 90% of all small business failures can be traced to poor management resulting from lack of knowledge. You need to be knowledgeable about

- Your profession (the clinical and non-clinical aspects).
- Your business (its products and services, priorities, financial requirements).
- Yourself (your strengths, weaknesses, goals, attitude to risk-taking).
- The marketplace (its relevance, size, new developments, socio-economic influences).
- The competition (who they are, what they offer).

Your knowledge and experience should become a springboard for innovation. Without this, you and your business cannot develop. The very knowledge and experience that helped get you where you are can paralyse your potential for progress. Your skills will include clinical skills as well as strategic skills. Strategic skills are those that enable you to take a broader view of

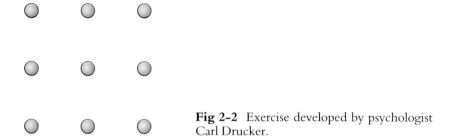

Fig 2-2 Exercise developed by psychologist Carl Drucker.

your business and to develop a vision and a goal. In short, to keep the vision on track.

To illustrate this, consider the following exercise developed by psychologist Carl Drucker. Look at the nine dots in Fig 2-2. The challenge is to connect all the dots with four straight lines without lifting your imaginary pen from the page once you have begun. The solution can be seen in Fig 2-3. To achieve the desired outcome you had to leave the imaginary box formed by the outline of the outer dots.

In their book *Think Out of the Box*, Vance and Deacon propose a series of questions to ask about any project. They call this "The Concept of Nine".

   1. Assess the way things are.
   2. Seek realistic thinking.
   3. See the vision.
   4. Ask why.
   5. Become change centred.
   6. Tap into ability.
   7. Ask how.
   8. Do not sanction incompetence.
   9. Implement and act.

Each member of your team has a MAP unique to him or her. It is your responsibility to bring these together before you embark on your journey and to remind everyone that the destination is the same.

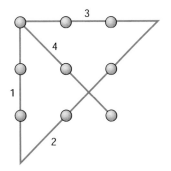

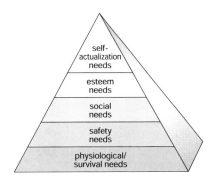

Fig 2-3 All the dots connected by four straight lines.

Fig 2-4 Maslow's hierarchy of needs.

Motivation

An understanding of human motivation is important in dentistry because it helps us better to understand our own behaviour, our team's behaviour and that of our patients. It is easy to forget sometimes that people can have a different set of priorities than our own and different degrees of motivation. We can talk about patients and members of our team and comment that they are "not motivated" without fully understanding and being aware of their circumstances.

Abraham Maslow is known for establishing a theory of motivation based on a hierarchy of needs. His work suggested that human beings are motivated by unsatisfied needs, and that certain lower needs need to be satisfied before higher needs can be satisfied (see Fig 2-4). In Maslow's model, needs are "prepotent"; a prepotent need is one that has the greatest influence over our actions. Everyone has a prepotent need, but the specific need will vary among individuals and we must remember to recognise this when we are working with people.

Physiological Needs

Our physiological needs are the very basic needs such as air, water, food, sleep, sex, etc. When these are not satisfied we may feel sickness, irritation, pain, discomfort. These feelings motivate us to alleviate them as soon as possible to establish homeostasis. Once they are alleviated, we may think about other things.

Safety Needs

Safety needs have to do with establishing stability and consistency in a chaotic world. These needs are mostly psychological in nature. We need the security of a home and family.

Love Needs

Love and "belongingness" are at the next level in the hierarchy. Humans have a desire to belong to groups: clubs, work groups, religious groups, family, gangs, etc. We need to feel loved by others, to be accepted by others. (Dental societies exist for that reason.)

Esteem Needs

There are two types of esteem needs. First is self-esteem, which results from competence or mastery of a task. Second, there is the attention and recognition that comes from others. All people in our society have a need or desire for self-respect, or self-esteem, and for the esteem of others. This is similar to the belongingness level. Wanting admiration, however, has to do with the need for power. For example, people who have all of their lower needs satisfied often drive very expensive cars because doing so raises their level of esteem. Satisfaction of the self-esteem need leads to feelings of self-confidence, worth, strength, capability and adequacy – of being useful and necessary in the world.

Self-actualisation

At the top of the pyramid, the need for self-actualisation is "the desire to become more and more what one is, to become everything that one is capable of becoming". People who have everything can maximise their potential.

Personal Qualities

Your business success will flow from your personal success. The two are inextricably linked. But the importance of personal factors is often ignored or given little importance in many business texts. All businesses start as a single thought – inspired by a personal vision, created by determination and managed with dedication. In other words, they are the physical manifestation of the elements of "self". The financial aspects of the business are process led and usually well defined. They are essential for commercial success, but they are irrelevant unless the business first achieves a status that merits or requires their application.

In 1990, Steven Covey published *The Seven Habits of Highly Effective People,* which has become one of the most successful books in history, with over 10 million copies sold. *The Seven Habits* teaches us that we must first master ourselves before being effective with others. It is the basis of success in the business of dentistry. The main principles behind each of these seven habits are summarised here.

Habit 1. Be proactive

Being proactive is about accepting responsibility for your own professional life. Our values are derived from experience (what happens to us), creativity (what we bring into existence) and attitude (our response to difficult circumstances). According to Covey, what matters most is how we *respond* to what we experience in life. We should take the initiative to make things happen – be proactive. The opposite of proactive is reactive – the tendency to react to environmental change.

Covey describes his concept by adopting the model shown in Fig 2-5. The inner circle is your circle of influence and the outer circle is the circle of concern. He suggests that there are some things that concern us that we cannot influence. But, there are many things that concern us that we can influence. Reactive people focus on their circle of concern. Proactive people focus on their circle of influence. Adopting a proactive stance also increases the diameter of your circle of influence, leaving less area of concern.

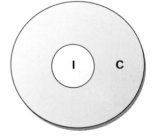

Fig 2-5 Covey's circles of influence (I) and concern (C).

Habit 2. Begin with the end in mind

According to Covey, "all things are created twice". We create them first in our minds, and then we work to bring them into physical existence. Many sportsmen and women use the principle – sometimes intuitively. I recall supervising my son in a shallow swimming pool when he was aged 7 years. He asked me if I could do an underwater somersault backwards. It was with some reluctance that I had to admit that this was not a skill I had acquired. He offered a solution. All I had to do was shut my eyes, see myself doing the said procedure, then open my eyes and just do it!

Remember the first rule of carpentry – "measure twice, cut once". It could just as easily be the first rule on clinical intervention. To introduce this philosophy into your personal and professional lives, develop a personal mission statement or philosophy. Make this the focus centre on your principles. And remember that you can always rely on your principles – they are deep and fundamental truths that should be the common denominator of your personal and professional life. If you find your actions are not congruent with your mission statement, you can create an affirmation to improve. An affirmation should have five ingredients: it should be personal, positive, present tense, visual, and emotional.

You can apply the principle to your practice. In Chapter 1, we discussed the importance of writing a practice mission statement. It gives a common

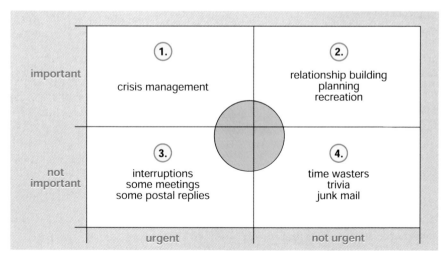

Fig 2-6 The time management matrix.

purpose to every employee in the practice and encourages the team to fulfil the aspirations of your business. In the 1960s, in the NASA headquarters, an employee in the catering department was asked by a visitor about her role in the organisation. She was swift in her reply – she was there to help put a man on the moon. She was right.

Habit 3. Put first things first

In any given day, the demands on our professional time (shown by the circle in Fig 2-6) will mean that we engage in activities that probably touch all four quadrants. Those in quadrant 1 are important and urgent. They are immediate and pressing problems: the compressor has stopped working; a patient requires treatment for prolonged haemorrhage; a child has arrived at the surgery with an avulsed tooth after a fall in the school playground. Such situations are easily recognised and usually highly visible, with known adverse consequences.

In quadrant 2, we encounter situations that are important but not necessarily urgent: the bank interest rate on the practice loan needs renegotiation; some referral letters (non-urgent) need to be written. Those activities that fit into quadrant 2 usually need a more proactive approach to make them happen. Habit 3 relies on habit 1 to affect it. Otherwise we may not get around to these activities at all. Covey suggests that we ask the question, "What one thing could you do in your personal and professional life that, if you did on a regular basis, would make a tremendous positive difference in your life?" The chances are that it is a quadrant 2 activity. We should aim to do it. Effective people spend most of their time in quadrant 2 and get results.

When we are in quadrant 3, we receive telephone calls, notification of meetings, new email arrives and the prompt box glows on the screen inviting us to "read it now?". The risk is that quadrant 3 activities may be perceived as quadrant 1 activities unless you are disciplined about working to your priorities not to the priorities or expectations of others.

Quadrant 4 is the so-called escape quadrant when we engage in activities that are neither urgent nor important. Try to minimise your activity in this quadrant and use the time saved for quadrant 2. Individuals who manage their life and their practice by crisis management will spend 90% of their time in quadrant 1 and need the other 10% in quadrant 4 to recover from the intense stress in the first quadrant.

To be effective, we need to stay clear of quadrants 3 and 4. It is the art of learning to say "no" to those activities that fall into these areas. Again, aim for quadrant 2 activities instead. By doing this you can shrink your quadrant 1 activities. Take the example of an automatic processor for developing radiographs. It is approaching the time when the solutions need renewal – it is important but it is not urgent. In other words, at this moment it is a quadrant 2 activity. If you proactive and change the solutions a crisis will not develop. If you are not proactive because there is no problem with image quality, and leave it alone, then suddenly the machine will "fail" and the radiographs will yield no diagnostic information. This happens in the middle of the morning on a day when you are short-staffed. Suddenly, it is important and urgent to get this machine working again and what should have been a quadrant 2 activity becomes a pressing quadrant 1 necessity that causes disruption to the working day.

Habit 4. Think "win–win"
"Win–win" is a philosophy and an attitude of mind that constantly seeks mutual benefit in all human interactions. In a "win–win" situation, outcomes and solutions are mutually beneficial and mutually satisfying.

In carrying out the business of dentistry we encounter a range of situations with patients and team members that reflect one of six interactive paradigms. These are:

1. "Win–win". In this scenario, people can seek mutual benefit and satisfaction in all human interactions.
2. "Win–lose". This is a competitive paradigm: if one person wins, then the other person loses. It reflects an authoritarian leadership style. To some extent we are all conditioned with this mentality. Two teams play in a match and we are told who has won and who has lost. Coming second is losing because we are conditioned to believe that "winner takes all". Covey states that the win–lose mentality obstructs the interdependence on which our lives depend.
3. "Lose–win". This has been described by some as the "doormat" paradigm. An individual will seek strength from popularity based on acceptance as a result of personal insecurity. Living this paradigm can also result in psychosomatic illness from repressed resentment.
4. "Lose–lose". This arises when two ego-driven people become obsessed with making the other person lose, even if it is at their own expense. I recall a situation when two dentists decided to go to court over a dispute concerning outstanding fees of £5,000 only to run up costs exceeding the amount that was in dispute. Each was determined to make the other

lose – despite sound advice to desist from the defence organisation.
5. "Win". The focus is solely on getting what one wants, regardless of the needs of others. In this paradigm, looking after "number one" is all that matters.
6. "No deal". In this paradigm, if a mutually beneficial, "win–win", solution cannot be found then the two parties agree to disagree agreeably – in other words, no deal. This approach is most realistic at the beginning of a business relationship. It is not an option in a continuing relationship.

Covey suggests that in "interdependent realities" we should think "win–win". The other paradigms may appear to be appropriate in the short-term but do not help to build relationships. In a competitive situation, where building a relationship is not important, "win–lose" may be appropriate, but it is unlikely in the people-centred business of dentistry.

The business of dentistry is about interdependency and relationship management, so – "win–win" should be the focus of our thinking. When there is a relationship of trust between dentist and patient, the emotional bank balances are high, and there is a greater probability of a successful and productive interaction. Within the practice team, you can facilitate the culture of "win–win" by:
• Seeing problems from the other point of view - in terms of the needs and concerns of the other party.
• Identifying the key issues and concerns (not positions) involved.
• Determining what results would help create a fully acceptable solution.
• Identifying new options to achieve those results.

A reward system is a key element in the "win–win" model. If you talk "win–win" you must walk "win–win". The temptation is to reward the outstanding performance of a few. If rewarded, the other team members will be losers, which goes against the "win–win" approach. Instead, try and develop individual achievable goals and team objectives to be rewarded.

Habit 5. Seek first to understand
Dentistry is a people (patient)-centred business. The fundamental tenet of any people-centred business is to put the individual first. This means understanding their attitudes, desires, needs and wants. Covey's interpretation of this is reflected in Habit 5 – "seek first to understand and then be understood".

This means that we need to develop the skills of empathic listening in a way

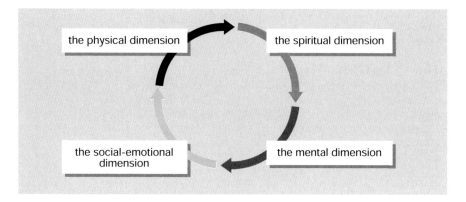

Fig 2-7 Covey's four-dimensional model.

that inspires openness and trust. Covey describes empathic listening as listening with our ears, our eyes and our heart. Empathic listening is listening with intent to understand the other person's frame of reference and feelings. As dentists, the danger is that we head for the logical side without first establishing character and building the relationship. Our responses to the concerns expressed by patients require empathic, logical-emotional responses. Covey uses an expression with which we can readily identify and one, which requires no explanation: "Diagnose before you prescribe."

Habit 6. Synergy
A simple definition of synergy is that "the whole is greater than the sum of its parts". Nowhere does synergy operate better than in the natural world. We can express the concept by an equation where $1 + 1 = 3$. The essence of synergy is to value differences – to respect them, to build on strengths, and to compensate for weaknesses. Covey suggests that, when properly understood, "synergy is the highest activity in all life". To create an environment in which it can flourish, use the principles outlined in habit 4 and the skills described in habit 5.

Habit 7. Sharpen the saw
Habit 7 is about preserving and enhancing your greatest asset in the business of dentistry: You. Sharpening the saw is an example of a quadrant 2 activity. Covey proposes a four-dimensional model (Fig 2-7) and cites this example. Suppose you came upon a lumberjack in the woods sawing down a tree. The lumberjack is exhausted from working long hours. You suggest they

take a break to sharpen the saw and therefore do what are doing more effectively. The lumberjack might reply, " I do not have time to sharpen the saw, I am too busy sawing!"

The Physical Dimension
The physical dimension is about looking after your physical body. This means sensible eating, allowing time for rest, relaxation and regular exercise and learning to manage stress. This is discussed later in this chapter.

The Spiritual Dimension
The spiritual dimension reflects your commitment and your values. It should be your source of inspiration and achievement.

The Mental Dimension
It is important keep your mind sharp by reading, writing, organising and planning. We should aim to read broadly and expose ourselves to great minds and leaders in thought. Covey's advice is that we should commit at least one hour to renewal in the first three dimensions: physical, spiritual and mental, on a daily basis.

The Social/Emotional Dimensions
The physical, spiritual and mental dimensions are closely related to habits 1, 2 and 3: personal vision, leadership and management.

The social/emotional dimensions focus on habits 4, 5 and 6: the principles of personal leadership, empathic communication and synergistic co-operation. Success in Habits 4, 5 and 6 is not primarily a matter of intellect, but emotion; it is highly related to our sense of personal security. Intrinsic security comes from within, from correct principles deep in our own mind and from living and practising with integrity, in which our daily habits reflect our deepest values. There is also intrinsic security that comes as a result of helping other people in a meaningful way, as our profession requires us to do.

It is interesting to compare Covey's perspective with that of The Pankey Institute in the USA. The core philosophy of the Institute states, "you cannot give your personal best if you are bored. You cannot give your personal best if you are lonely and unappreciated. The productive, happy life contains a balance of work, recreation, loving relationships, and spiritual pursuits".

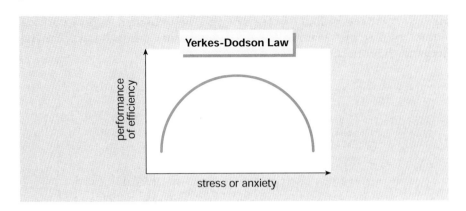

Fig 2-8 The relationship between stress and performance.

Stress and Performance

Stress is a state of imbalance. It was defined by Hans Selye, a notable researcher in psychosomatic medicine, as "the non-specific response of the body to any demand made upon it". Understanding how stress affects us is an important part of self-management and it is the key to developing successful coping strategies. If you are not able to handle the stress of the business of dentistry, then your judgement will be clouded and your performance will suffer.

Robert Yerkes and John Dodson first investigated the relationship between stress and performance in 1908. They noted that stress and performance were linked in a curvilinear way – in the form of an inverted U (Fig 2-8). In the first part of the curve, stress actually improves our efficiency. But, past a certain point, the reverse occurs: ongoing stress impairs our effectiveness. In fact, working longer or harder beyond that point is not only unproductive, it is *counter*productive. It could be looked upon as a variation of the law of diminishing returns.

Research suggests that almost half of all adults suffer adverse affects due to stress and it is known that dentistry is perceived as one of the most stressful occupations. The management of stress in the practice environment has important implications for the business of dentistry. In one study it was concluded that almost 60% of staff absences were attributed to psychological problems that were stress-related. Many dentists work long hours, but very few people can put in more than ten hours a day (or fifty hours a week) and still be productive. After that, not only does everything take longer, but we become tired and inefficient.

Here is an extract from the writings of Dr David Posen, a highly respected author, speaker, physician, athlete, and musician in Canada. It is reproduced here with his kind and personal permission.

> "When I was in general practice and reached a critical mass of patients to see, phone calls to return, and paperwork to deal with, the word that flashed through my mind was "ENOUGH" - like a big neon sign. I'd pause, sit down with my nurse and start delegating like crazy - finally making decisions I had been putting off for days. The pile of charts on my desk would fade within minutes, leaving me a manageable workload again, and a great sense of relief.
>
> "Enough" is another word we should add to our work-life balance vocabulary. The workday is getting longer and faster and more open-ended. To get control of this situation we need to start asking, How much is enough? How much is enough time spent at work? How much is enough achievement and success? How much is enough money?"

According to David Posen, we are responsible for a lot of our own stress. He draws the following conclusions from his vast experience:

- Most of the stress that most of us have is self-generated. We create most of our own distress.
- We have more control than we think. But, too often, we do not use it.
- There is no silver bullet or quick fix for relieving stress (although exercise and relaxation techniques come pretty close). To master stress we have to change.
- Stress mastery is as much a mind set as it is a collection of tools and strategies. It is the knowledge and confidence that, whatever happens, we will be able to handle it.

The business of dentistry will challenge you from time to time, and being able to handle a situation is a critical success factor frequently omitted.

Further Reading

Covey SR. The Seven Habits of Highly Effective People. New York: Simon & Schuster, 1990.

Maslow A. Motivation and Personality. New York: Harper, 1954.

Posen D. The Principles of Stress. www.davidposen.com.

Vance M, Deacon, D. Think Out of the Box. Franklin Lakes, NJ: Career Press, 1997.

Whitman H. Success is Within You. New York: Doubleday & Co., 1956.

Yerkes RM, Dodson JD. The relation of strength of stimulus to rapidity of habit-formation. J Compar Neurol Psychol 1908;18:459-482.

Chapter 3
Patient–centred Care

The blend of art and science that is dentistry can make us forget that the business of dentistry is a "people business" and that we should adopt a patient-centred approach in all that we do. Patient-centred care is about relationship management. The relationship between dentist and patient should be one built on trust. "Technique and technology are important", says Tom Peters, "but adding trust is the issue of the decade."

In the July 2000 NHS Plan, a patient-centred service was amongst the leading pledges of the government. A briefing paper from the King's Fund noted that :

> "Patient-centred care demands that health professional do not simply diagnose and treat illness as a technical exercise in problem solving but that they work in partnership with patients and carers – listening to their concerns, responding to their anxieties, acknowledging their values and respecting multiple demands on their lives. It means that each consultation between a health professional and a patient is an exercise in partnership, with equal power rather than one dominating the other."

The sentiment would apply equally when seen from a business perspective.

Relationship Management

Relationship management is all about communication and delivering and exceeding the patient's expectations. We know that effective communication skills are amongst the most valued skills from a patient's perspective and there have been studies undertaken to try to identify what elements of the interpersonal relationship most matter to patients. The identified factors were:
• being greeted warmly

- being listened to
- receiving clear explanations
- being given reassurance
- having confidence in the health professional's abilities
- being able to express concerns and fears
- being respected
- being given enough time during the visit
- consideration being made of their personal context
- concern being given for the patient as a person

The 2 June 2002 Business Section of the *The Sunday Times* carried an article by Maria Yapp about high flyers in business. She quoted from the work of leading business psychologists and concluded that, in addition to core capabilities, "high flyers have emotional intelligence – superior 'soft' skills – which they use to form and manage relationships. They are skilled in negotiation and leadership, demonstrating enhanced ability in the way they motivate and deal with others".

Dealing with people can be difficult, and dealing with difficult people is often impossible. The reason, according to Dale Carnegie, is that when dealing with people we must remember that we are not dealing with creatures of logic but with creatures of emotion.

Satisfaction and Loyalty

In the past there has been some assumptions in business that:
- it is sufficient simply to satisfy your customer.
- the time and energy involved to create *absolute* satisfaction are not worth it
- efforts at delivering satisfaction should be based on lowest common denominators, i.e. "base-line expectations".

These assumptions do not accurately reflect what is known about relationship management in business today. The relationship between customer satisfaction and loyalty (retention) is not a linear one. It reflects the skewed relationship that is Pareto's principle (see Chapter 1). The level of satisfaction that produces an exponential rise in loyalty (increased loyalty) comes from the last 20% of the effort to deliver that satisfaction. This relationship is shown in Fig 3-1.

The shaded area is the "zone of defection" where the patient could easily

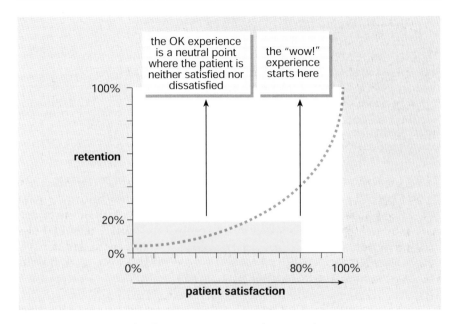

Fig 3-1 The relationship between patient satisfaction and retention.

seek care elsewhere. This zone gets narrower as the relationship between dentist and patient matures and goodwill is added to the emotional bank account. Satisfaction because a cumulative experience.

The challenge of delivering the "wow!" experience is that it gets harder each time you interact with the patient. Today's "wow!" factor is tomorrow's baseline expectation. For example, I recall a patient who was telephoned after the uneventful extraction of a lower third molar. The patient was delighted to receive the call and could not thank me enough. Two weeks later, after the extraction of the opposite molar, I failed to call the patient during the evening as I was attending a lecture. On his return to the practice the following week for a review appointment, the patient thanked me again for calling him the first time, but remarked that he was disappointed not to receive a call from me on the second occasion. Apparently he had planned to go out but thought he would stay in as he expected me to telephone. I had delivered the "wow!" experience on the first occasion but fallen short of the expectation on the second. From "wow!" to a veiled complaint in less than ten working days!

Delivering Satisfaction

Many studies looking into patient satisfaction with dental care identify five generic themes. These are:
- technical competence
- interpersonal factors
- convenience
- costs
- facilities.

The results have been contradictory because of demographic variables, such as:

Age Patients of 60 years of age or more tend to be more satisfied with their dental care than younger patients, but less satisfied with the communication process.

Gender Women express greater levels of satisfaction with dental care than men. One reason may be their greater exposure to the service, which in turn could have a moderating effect on their expectations.

Economic status Patients from low-income groups have different attitudes to their dental health and seek care less frequently.

Previous dental experiences Patients whose previous experience of their dentist has been positive report higher levels of satisfaction. They will forgive the occasional episode of poor performance, attributing this to "uncontrollable" or "sporadic" elements.

Regular v. irregular attendance Some studies have indicated no difference between the two groups but others have suggested that there is a positive correlation between frequency of attendance and satisfaction.

Anxiety levels It has been demonstrated that patients who exhibit high levels of anxiety tend to be more dissatisfied with their care than their less-anxious counterparts.

Expectation and Experience

What should patients expect from their healthcare provider? It has been suggested that the key elements are:

Access Patient care when it is needed and whenever it is needed. This includes access to Internet- and telephone-based services for advice.

Personalised care Patients should be treated as individuals, offered choices and have an opportunity to indicate preferences.

Control The system can take control but only if the patient consents.

Information Patients can know what they wish to know. Their clinical records are theirs.

Transparency Confidentiality is assured, but patients should have access to anything and everything about their care and treatment that they wish to have access to.

Science Patients have the right to care based on the best available scientific knowledge – in other words, evidence-based dentistry.

Safety Patients should not be harmed in their environment.

Anticipation Anticipate patient needs by giving proactive help that goes beyond just reactive care.

Value Care should not waste the patient's time and money.

Co-operation Teams that provide care should co-ordinate their efforts so as to create a seamless experience.

Many of these themes echo the principles of clinical governance. A customer's expectation of service quality is measured on two levels: the level of service representing a blend of what customers believe can be and should be provided and the minimum level of service customers are willing to accept (see Fig 3-2). The difference between experience and expectation is a measure of the dissatisfaction a patient has with the provider of that service (either from your practice or from you as an individual practitioner). In the former

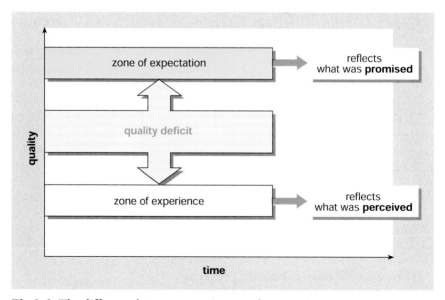

Fig 3-2 The difference between experience and expectation.

case, patients may opt to seek their care elsewhere, and in the latter case, they may request to see another dentist in the same practice.

Retention

Acquiring new patients is expensive. Retaining patients is much less so. It has been suggested that, on average, it costs five times as much to get a new patient as it does to retain an existing one.

In his book *Customers for Life* Carl Sewell advises on how to ensure customer retention. In summary, he states that we should:
- ask them what they want and give it to them each time
- under-promise and over-deliver
- show people respect irrespective of their socio-economic background
- measure everything
- invite complaints and deal with them effectively.

This list accords closely with other views. For example, under-promise and over-deliver is another way of expressing the satisfaction model shown in Fig 3-2. The point about effective handling of complaints is particularly interesting. We all make mistakes and there is a natural tendency to avoid a thorough investigation of them on the basis that you cannot please all of the people all of the time. But, we also know that if one patient complains about something the chances are that others have thought about it as well (it has been estimated that for every customer who complains twenty-six do not).

The way in which complaints are handled is crucial in any business. Research suggests that over 95% of customers will forgive you if their concerns are handled quickly. Of these, around 20% will tell others how great you are at solving problems. Studies of customer behaviour indicate that when asked why they changed from one service provider to another almost half the customers mention poor service as a reason for change. In comparison, only 8% mention the technical aspects of the product, and only 8% mention price. Carl Sewell's findings (Fig 3-3) suggest that the percentage leaving because of poor service is higher still: 68% of customers leaving do so because of what they perceive as an indifferent attitude on the part of the service provider and a further 9% make up their minds on the basis of the poor quality of the encounter.

Others cite similar ratios. Professor Len Berry is one of the leading authorities in the fields of retailing and service quality. He investigated the 68% who leave because of poor service in more detail and identified, through factor

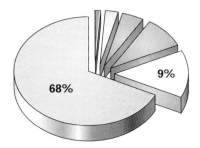

Fig 3-3 The reasons customers leave.

analysis, that the causes fall into the five categories: reliability, assurance, empathy, responsiveness and tangibles. These are discussed in more detail in Chapter 4.

Patient Referrals

New patient referrals are the lifeblood of any practice. Satisfied patients generate referrals. Research carried out by the US Office of Consumer Affairs shows that satisfied customers are likely to pass on their good impressions of a company to five other people. In contrast, dissatisfied customers are likely to tell at least eleven others. This observation has become known anecdotally as the 5/11 Rule, although it is recognised that the ratios can vary from one type of service to another. The important point here is to recognise the leveraged relationship.

In *Thriving on Chaos* Tom Peters writes that we should "consider every customer to be a potential lifelong customer, generating word-of-mouth referrals" and in so doing emphasises the relationship with the customer over a period of time. The outcome of this relationship will be a growth in word-of-mouth recommendations. This subject is covered in Chapter 6.

The "Credibility Factor"

Your patients must find you to be competent, caring and credible. You earn credibility when people believe you can do what you say. You can help build credibility by:
- demonstrating that your clinical skills are up to date (providing solutions to your patients' problems)
- showing that you care about your patients.
- showing that you care about the reputation of your practice.

Table 3-1. **Dentist- or patient-centred practice?**

Dentist–centred practice	Patient-centred practice
Nothing has changed. The environment is exactly the same and change is resisted. It is very much business as usual. Yesterday's strategy continues to prevail. There is a view that change is often unnecessary and always a threat.	The patient is now a sophisticated dental consumer. Change is inevitable and presents new opportunities. There is recognition that change is inevitable and should benefit the patients.
Patients get in the way of running a practice. They are difficult, complaining and don't understand how hard it is for us to run the practice.	We need to identify what our patients want and adapt our services and facilities to meet those desires.
Surgery hours should be based on what is convenient for the dentists.	Surgery hours should reflect the needs and demands of the marketplace.
It is expensive to run a practice. We should minimise costs. There is no need to spend unnecessarily. There is under-investment in the business.	We should move with the times and develop new services to reflect what patients demand. There is willingness to invest in good equipment and a pleasant waiting room environment.
The dentists always know best. A paternalistic view on patient care prevails.	Involve the patients in decision making. Empower them to decide for themselves.
Complaints are seen as a reflection of an ungrateful patient.	Complaints are seen as an opportunity to improve the standard of care to patients.
Patient satisfaction measures are not used – on the basis that patients cannot be objective about what they perceive as quality care.	Patient opinions are sought and it is recognised that qualitative measures of satisfaction are as important as quantitative measures.

- displaying certificates of courses attended and qualifications obtained.
- displaying practice achievements (awards, etc.)
- inference (a practice website, for example, shows that you keep up with the times).

Planning for a Patient-centred Practice

So what makes a practice patient-centred? The key differences between dentist-centred and patient-centred practices are shown in Table 3-1. Here are some "dos" and "don'ts" about planning for a patient-centred practice.

Do

Make patients feel welcome and wanted Treat all patients as though they are guests in your own home. Use all opportunities to communicate, such as welcome packs, information leaflets, email messages.

Make the practice welcoming and inviting Ensure that customer-contact employees are people-friendly, and train them on the importance and perspective of customers. Establish speedy response times for the telephone, postal enquiries, and email.

Facilitate access to your services Have a transparent pricing policy. Provide accurate and up-to-date information about your services. Obtain an unbiased assessment of your literature readability and availability.

Participate in post-treatment communications Communication with your patients should be ongoing. Mail them reminders, newsletters, advice and information leaflets, satisfaction surveys.

Invite feedback from your patients Anticipate and prevent problems for customers before they happen. Listen to patients to learn about their concerns. When problems occur, respond promptly, and keep the patient informed during any resolution process. Do not just solve the problem – exceed the expectation. Positive feedback will inform you what they like about you and is always welcome. And it will help you accept the negative comments more easily.

Exceed the baseline expectation Each time a patient arrives at your practice, they have a certain expectation. The challenge is to identify it and exceed it. If the expectation is unrealistic, the challenge then is to make it more realistic before trying to find ways of exceeding it. In a new practice, you may introduce new techniques and facilities into your practice and expect your patients to give you an immediate response. Somehow this never seems to happen in the timeframe you anticipate.

Don't

Ignore the views of your team Expenditure on the team is an investment not an unnecessary expense. Motivating, coaching and managing your staff are probably some of your toughest challenges in general dental practice today. Remember that a lack of morale and motivation can rapidly erode profits.

Confuse likelihood with reality Remember the successful entrepreneur lives in a world of likelihood. (As an accountant, my co-author would like to take this opportunity to remind readers that expenditure takes place in the world of reality!)

Stand still Where your business is today is down to what you did yesterday. Times change. Yesterday's success was based on yesterday's strategy and that is no guarantee that tomorrow will be the same.

Features and Benefits

"Ask them what and give it to them each time" is Carl Sewell's way of delivering and exceeding the customer's expectation. But do we really know what our patients want? It may not be what you and I think it should be.

The example quoted by American management guru Theodore Levitt involves the purchase of a drill. The drill is purchased not for its physical qualities, but to make holes. Consider the purchase of an expensive motor car. Whether we like it or not, the image and status associated with Porsche, Ferrari and Aston Martin are key factors in the purchase of the vehicle. The features of these cars such as build quality, engine design and thoroughbred pedigree are often used to justify the purchase rather than inspire it in the first place. As dentists, it is easy to focus on what we do – the technical aspects, the science and the excitement of new technologies. What patients are seeking are the benefits that stem from those features.

Consider the features of modern endodontic techniques, for example. Preparation times are reduced by the use of nickel-titanium instruments of greater taper and ultrasonic irrigation is an efficient way to irrigate the root canal system. Thermoplastic obturation techniques are quicker than conventional multi-point condensation techniques. The benefits to the patient may include less time in the chair, more predictable results in less time and fewer appointments. Always aim to translate the features of your practice into how the patients are likely to benefit from them and highlight these in your discussions with them.

Further Reading

Berry L. On Great Service. New York: The Free Press, 1995.

Peters T. Liberation Management. London: Pan, 1992.

Peters T. The Pursuit of Wow!: Every Person's Guide to Topsy-Turvy Times. New York: Random House, Inc., 1994.

Peters T. Thriving on Chaos: Handbook for a Management Revolution. London: Pan, 1987.

Sewell C. Customers for Life. New York: Doubleday Currency, 1990.

Chapter 4
Perception is Reality

Meeting patients' expectations is an essential link in the service-profit chain. When a new patient arrives at your practice, she or he will have prior expectations. These may relate to the way they are greeted, the environment, the range of services you provide, the fees and the way they are treated. As they approach your premises, those expectations are in a state of flux influenced by everything going on around them. This engagement of the senses is what perception is about and it helps to create the reality in the patient's mind and it plays an important part in remodelling expectation.

But, it is not always as easy as it sounds. The reason is that perception is affected by so many variables and they can be different for different people. And when they are the same, different people attach different value to them.

As Colin Cherry puts it in *On Human Communication*:

> "though many different pairs of people may say 'the same thing' (linguistically) on different occasions in conversation, each occasion, as an event, is observably different in many aspects from the others; such differences depend upon people's accents, their past experiences, their present states of mind, the environment, the future consequences of interpreting the message, knowledge of each other, and many other factors …"

Whether we like it or not, we have all been conditioned to interpret visual images in certain ways. For example, if food on a plate looks attractive, then the association is that it must taste good. There are few absolute truths – it is all down to what you see and what conclusions you draw from what you see.

The Psychology of Perception

The science behind managing the perception is psychology. "Spin doctoring" is the popular term to describe the work of those who apply the psychology of human perceptions in their work. It is a sophisticated form of marketing. It is a great pity that a valuable tool has achieved notoriety because of the way it has come to be used. "Spin doctor, heal thyself" would not be inappropriate advice to the industry. For this reason, the word is used with caution and relates to the psychology of perception – not its perceived meaning. The irony will not be lost on readers.

To be effective, spin has to be invisible. Timothy Bewes, author of *Cynicism and Postmodernity*, writes: "the moment when we become aware of the existence of spin is the moment of its disappearance. Effective spin requires a general unawareness of its existence." The power of positive perceptions underpins word-of-mouth marketing; it leads to recommendations and helps to build successful businesses.

Your Professional Image

How we look, dress, act and speak all contribute to our image. Psychologists refer to it as pattern recognition – we "template match". When new patients enter your practice, they template match from the moment of arrival. Ask yourself the question: does your practice image reflect the typical template or there is something about it that makes you different? Is there anything you could do to break the mould and alter the perception – something akin to the "wow!" factor?

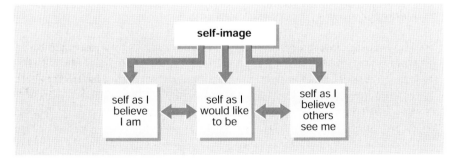

Fig 4-1 Self-image and self-esteem.

The Greek philosopher Epictetus probably never thought of himself as a spin doctor. He was, however, acutely aware of the psychology of perception. He taught his pupils "first to know who you are, then adorn yourself accordingly". So, before you look at your practice, look at yourself.

Self-image is where it starts. Dimbleby and Burton in their book *More Than Words* proposed the model shown in Fig 4-1. There is a relationship between self-image and self-esteem. The more positive one's self-image, the higher one's self-esteem. Self-image is connected also with communication performance. For example, if we believe we are ugly, we may expect to be rejected. We may as a result enter into communication expecting rejection and thus present ourselves in a way, which actually invites rejection – the so-called self-fulfilling prophecy. We are also likely to seek from others confirmation that our self-image is accurate. Thus, if we see ourselves as winners, so will others and, as a result we may well turn out to be winners; if we see ourselves as losers, then losers is what we may become.

Anecdotal evidence suggests that many dentists do not relish the thought of discussing costs of treatment. Many writers in the field of practice management describe a phenomenon where the brain suggests the correct fee for a procedure but the mouth utters a lesser one – the so-called oro-fiscal drag! (In fact, my co-author refers to it in Chapter 7.) This observation is based partly on fear of rejection and any communication with patients on the subject could turn out to be a self-fulfilling prophecy.

Choice of clothing can also affect the patient's perception. Clothing influences first impressions. The white coat has become a symbol of the health professional, but these conventions are not as rigid as they once were. Style and cleanliness in clothing may be more important and indicate adherence to traditional values of hygiene and sterility.

So who is going to take responsibility for your image? Only *you* can and you must. It is an essential discipline in all aspects of the business of dentistry, including clinical dentistry. Self-monitoring is the term that has been coined by psychologists to express the extent to which a person notices the self-presentation of others and uses that information to guide their own self-presentation. People who score highly on their ability to self-monitor are better able to change their behaviour to suit the situation or audience – and are known to perform better.

The Halo and Horn Effects

The assumptions that we make are known as the "halo effect". This has been defined as bias created by an observer's tendency to rate, perhaps unintentionally, certain objects or persons in a manner that reflects what was previously anticipated. For example, people with glasses and high foreheads are frequently thought of as intelligent – even if we may not have direct evidence of this. The "horn effect" refers to the same phenomenon, but relates to undesirable characteristics. Anecdotal evidence suggests that we frequently judge (or rather misjudge) our patients in this way, making assumptions about their ability to afford treatment and their motivation, without having the evidence. By being aware of the tendency, it is possible to override it.

The Weighted Averaging Effect

We know that our judgements of other people are weighted averages of the information we have about them. In reaching decisions about our patients and their personalities and motivation towards dental health, we tend to take everything we know about them, but give some information a greater weight, and then produce an average of the information we have. Negative information will generally be given more weight than positive information. The same process takes place when patients look at us – they make the same weighted judgement errors.

The "Primacy" Effect

The "primacy" effect is a psychological term that means that when presented with a bunch of information, what we remember most often is that which entered the mind first. In other words, first impressions count. What could be more important in a patient-centred business? The primacy effect reflects the weighted average phenomenon: the information we obtain first is weighted more heavily than the rest because it is assumed to be more important.

The "Recency" Effect

It is also generally accepted, somewhat paradoxically, that if there is a significant time lag between the first piece of information and the next, then the last piece of information will carry more weight. This is known as the "recency" effect.

The notion of the primacy effect that "first impressions count" was challenged in a televised experiment carried out on the BBC Television programme *Tomorrow's World* in March 1995. In this experiment viewers saw a young man being interviewed for a job as an ambulance driver. He began by saying that he had been in the army medical corps and gave some description of his experience there. He ended by saying that he had not stayed long in any job since leaving the army. This was broadcast in one part of the country. In another part, viewers saw the facts presented in reverse order, i.e. he stated first that he had not held any job long after leaving the army. In the latter broadcast 54% of viewers voted that he had made a favourable impression in comparison to only 45% in the first broadcast – which seems to suggest that last impressions count.

Stereotyping

Stereotypes are generalisations about what people in a particular group are like. The social identity theory has been very influential in European psychology and suggests that we need to create social maps, which we do by grouping, and then uphold values and traditions of our own groups relative to other groups. The groups can be defined on any number of criteria but the common ones are:
- gender
- race
- occupation
- age.

In general practice, patients tend to be identified within these broad categories but also within sub-categories according to the structure of the practice. Patients may be labelled as either NHS (further divided into fee-paying and exempt) or private, and associations are made between job status and affordability. The managing director is one stereotype – she or he must be well paid, able to afford private care, be highly motivated towards oral health, and so on. Psychologists have suggested there is a tendency for us all to lean towards stereotyping, so we must learn to inhibit the "automatically activated stereotype" to become non-prejudicial.

We must remember that patients also display stereotype tendencies towards dentists. If the perceptions are negative (as they often are), the real challenge is to break the stereotype mould – but that is not easily done. Consider a typical remark made by a patient and one that many dentists have heard on numerous occasions in one form or another: "I hope I do not have to see you again too soon. I do not know why I say that. You have never hurt me, but you know what I mean." The patient is recalling information that is consistent with their pre-existing stereotype rather than information that is not consistent – as evidenced by the comment "I do not know why I say that. *You* have never hurt me." It can take time to change the image of the stereotype that is "the dentist" and one way to go about it is to borrow some ideas from the image-makers and the brand creators.

Branding

The concept of branding has become relevant in the business of dentistry because of new entrants into the business. Many of the dental bodies corporate are branded and are aware that branding makes a difference to the way people make choices about products and services. James Hull and Associates (now part of Integrated Dental Holdings), Whitecross Dental Care, Oasis, Boots and Dentics (now part of Dencare) are just some examples.

We should remember that whilst patient choice may be driven by utilitarian motives that include economic and functional value, it is influenced greatly by psychological values – so called self-expressive motives. The brand is the visual, emotional, rational and cultural image that we as consumers associate with a company or a product. It is important to stress the value of these associations because this is exactly what happens when a patient arrives at your practice. The psychology of perception is all about associations. In some cases, the associations have taken over – the brand name "Hoover" is often used in place of the generic "vacuum cleaner".

If you build associations, then you build the brand and it comes to reflect how you position yourself in the marketplace. When we think Volvo, we might think safety. When we think Nike, we might think of Michael Jordan or the phrase "Just Do It". Branding helps to enhance the value and satisfaction we get from a product or service. A good example of this brand strength is Coca-Cola. In blind tests involving Coke and rival colas, Coke did not finish first in the ratings. In other tests, when brand names were made known to the participants, Coke invariably finished first.

Your practice is already a brand. You are a unique brand as far as your patients are concerned. What we have always called "goodwill" is our intangible asset. It has value – industry calls it brand value. Coca-Cola is valued in excess of $45 billion and Gillette, by comparison, at $10 billion. Fairly tangible, don't you think?

We have never had to think of ourselves in this way, but the dental market-place is changing and we need to be proactive to stay competitive. Branding the practice will help to:

- Separate you from your competitors.
- Create and enhance your perceived value.
- Launch new products and services.
- Support your practice at times when the profession receives negative press coverage.
- Sustain your practice when faced with price-led competition.
- Establish your identity.

What makes up a brand identity?

Your brand identity is your public image. It is a connecting mechanism between your practice and your individual patients. A good brand identity will help you stand out from your competitors and consciously and sub-consciously draws patients to your practice. According to Eric Marder of Eric Marder Associates, one of the leading marketing consultancies, brand-ing is the "collateral information that has been attached to the brand by exter-nal symbols: words, pictures and music". This collateral information comes in two parts – the "label" and the "fable". The intrinsic feature of the label is the brand name. The fable is the extrinsic element attached by the imagery of advertising. The fable sends out the social messages. "Buy brand X of body spray and you will become more attractive to the opposite sex" is just one example. You need only to look at some of the leading women's and men's lifestyle magazines to see examples of how some dentists present these social messages.

To put it another way, your practice logo, the staff uniforms, the sign on the building are all part of your "label". In time, these come to mean something to your patients and what it comes to mean is the "fable" part of the con-cept. Do not underestimate the power of the label. It has been shown that consumers show preferences on their perception of labels even when the products they describe are identical.

Your brand identity will be built from:

- your brand name
- your logo
- your market position
- the brand associations
- your brand personality.

A good brand name gives a good first impression and evokes positive associations with the brand. A positioning statement tells the patient about your philosophy of care, what benefits it provides and why it is better than the competition. Brand personality essentially adds emotion and culture and "fable" to the identity.

Brand associations are the attributes that patients think of when they hear or see your practice brand name – this is what drives growth in business.

Creating your brand
Branding is not just for big business. It should be the starting point in any marketing strategy. The creative process often starts with a logo. But remember that there is more to your brand than just your logo – or your practice colour scheme or the design theme inside your practice. These features are all graphical parts of your brand identity. They are incorrectly and narrowly referred to as "branding". Branding is more than that; it is the sum total of patient experiences and perceptions, some of which you can influence, and some you cannot.

To help you to create your brand:

You must have a vision for your practice. (Understand your vision and objectives. Involve your team and make sure they understand them as well. To succeed, your branding program must have their understanding and support – and must serve the practice's objectives.)

Look at the competition. (Evaluate their marketing communications. For example, look at the corporate sector and try to determine the range of "values" that are associated with the larger groups. Look at how they position themselves. This can tell you what territory they are claiming and how strongly. It can also tell you what they are not claiming where there might be a gap. Gaps are anything but space – they are opportunities.)

Find out what your patients expect and what matters to them, and try and determine how you are rated on these values.

Develop your strategy. (Your desired position in the market should be achievable, compelling, likeable, long-term and sustainable.)

Get team commitment across the practice.

Develop an integrated approach to all marketing communications. (There must be continuity and consistency in all that you do.)

Measure outcomes. (Try and get feedback by setting up a response system to measure effectiveness of your efforts. Ask new patients why they have chosen to come to your practice.)

Continuously evaluate and improve. (Make changes as needed, but be patient and let your marketing programmes build your brand.)

Strength and Stature

Brand building then is about:
- knowledge (awareness, experience and understanding on the part of the patient)
- esteem (your reputation and the level of patient respect for your practice)
- relevance (your efforts must be meaningful to patients and important to *them*)
- differentiation (the elements which make your practice unique).

The *stature* of your brand is derived from the knowledge and esteem elements. Your brand *strength* comes from the differentiation and relevance elements.

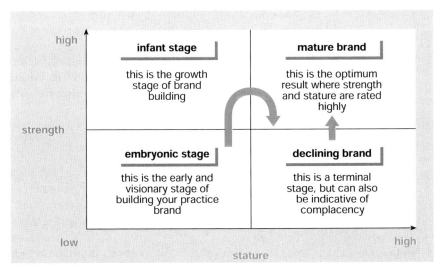

Fig 4-2 Brand building.

Typically, brand building follows the path shown by the curved arrow in Fig 4-2. Complacency can precipitate a rapid decline, and it is important to take corrective action before the damage is done so as to regain the mature status where strength and statute remain highly rated. All businesses are prone to this. One recent example has been Marks and Spencer, where the declining brand had to be rescued to achieve its former status.

Your practice's future is built on its past. The same is true of brands. Eric Marder's Image Principle states "It is easier to give a brand the right image in the first place than to change a wrong image once it has taken hold". This is where your marketing communications and the marketing mix come into the equation.

Your environment says something about you – the choice of colour, texture, lighting and ambient design gives your practice a certain image. In other words, the environment can enhance or, if poorly designed, detract from the image of the brand. Together with price and familiarity it can add what Marder calls "a positive or negative increment" to the perception of the brand.

Useful hints and tips
Here are ten practical pointers to think about if you are considering changing your practice image:

1. Do not undervalue your label. It is what makes you successful and it is why patients come to you. Build on this strength.
2. If members of your professional team have not been with you for very long, remember that they are the ones who will need the additional props of brand building to compensate for the fact that they have yet to establish their label.
3. Look at your practice environment. Is it in keeping with your style of practice and is it in keeping with the trends in your locality? The environment is a prop for those who have yet to establish themselves with their patients. In time, it may become less important or may play a supportive rather than a prime role in building the brand.
4. Monitor the wider marketplace to get a feel for the standard that may be expected by your patients.
5. Create consistency within your image. For example, a high-tech environment and poor-quality stationery are sending a mixed message to your patients.

6. Pay attention to details like colours, textures and lighting when designing the environment.
7. Consider a change of uniform for the team. It is a good way of communicating to everyone that the image of the practice is changing.
8. Remember that change need not be costly. Subtle changes can add significant positive "increments" to the perception.
9. Do not rush. Remember it is far easier to give a brand the right image from the outset rather than try and change it once it has taken hold.
10. When you know what image you want to portray, create your mission statement and design your logo in a way that reflects your intentions.

Interpersonal communication
Branding and marketing strategy rely on effective communication. The classic model that is often used to introduce the subject of communication is shown in Fig 4-3. It suggests that there is a start point and an end point in all communication. This may be true in some dentist–patient interactions, but often what happens is cyclical in nature. In person-to-person communication, the encoding process is performed by the motor skills of the source – the vocal mechanism. In a telephone conversation, the telephone electronics act as the encoder – turning your sounds into electrical impulses.

The message is the substance of the communication process. Just as a source needs an encoder to translate her purposes into a message, so the receiver

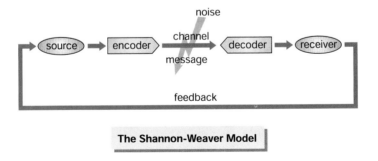

The Shannon-Weaver Model

Fig 4-3 The classic communication model.

needs a decoder to retranslate. Decoding then is about interpretation. Communication breakdowns arise because the processes of encoding and decoding are not always predictable. Misunderstandings arise when the intended meaning and perceived meaning are different.

These can arise for a number of reasons:

Attitude differences. (If you are aware of an attitude that might, in the presence of any given receiver, arouse hostility, then you will be aware that it would be appropriate to conceal that attitude. Clearly, if you are unaware of the attitude, then you will not attempt to conceal it and your communication may fail as a result, despite whatever other skills you may have.)

The choices of communication channel (Some messages may be more effective in the non-verbal channel than in the verbal channel. The use of clinical photographs and models is far more effective at explaining complex procedures than words can ever be.)

The complexity of the subject matter. (It is very likely that the patient knows far less about the procedures we perform than we do. Words and phrases that have obvious meaning to us can mean different things to different patients. The story of a patient who commented "it may not be vital to you but it is to me" was allegedly in direct response to a dentist explaining that a tooth was "non-vital".)

Social and cultural variables. (These influence the context in which words and actions can be interpreted.)

In K R Kulich's study of interpersonal skills in the dentist–patient relationship, a group of patients rated the quality of interpersonal skills to be at least as important as clinical skills amongst their ideal characteristics of a dentist. The attributes were, in order:
- contact with patients
- communication skills
- empathy
- manual skills
- theoretical knowledge.

In Corah and colleagues' report on "behaviour that reduces patient anxiety and increases satisfaction", patients frequently recommend dentists who:
- Give initial explanations of what is going to happen during a dental procedure.
- Give an in-process explanation to let the patient know what is happening as it is going on.

- Instruct the patient to be calm.
- Warn the patient about pain when it is likely to occur.
- Verbally support the patient.
- Try to give the patient ways of looking at the procedure in a less-threatening fashion and provide coaching to make them believe it is not as bad as they expect it to be.
- Provide distraction of attention and try to communicate in ways that builds trust.

Non-verbal Communication

Non-verbal communication is the valve that regulates the flow of verbal communication. It is a more powerful and more effective communication tool than words alone. In fact, no matter how carefully the words are chosen in face-to-face communication, if the paralinguistic cues (which reflect someone's emotional state) differ, the message will be insincere. Letters of complaint from patients about their dentist rarely go into detail about unsatisfactory treatment but will often cite the insincerity of the dentist's apology, which suggests that the patient has spotted the inconsistency between the substance of the message and the style of its delivery. The point is best illustrated in an old Chinese proverb: "Beware the man whose belly does not move when he laughs." It has been suggested that interpersonal liking is made up of three elements in different proportions, with facial expressions being the primary source of information (see Fig 4-4).

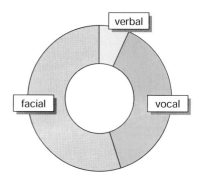

Fig 4-4 Interpersonal likeability.

Table 4-1. **Categories of personal space**

Degree of intimacy	Distance
Intimate distance	Ranges from direct physical contact to approximately 50 cm. It is usually for individuals with whom we have an intimate relationship. This is also the working zone in all clinical dental procedures.
Casual distance	Ranges from just under 1 metre to 1.5 metres and involves individuals who are comfortable with each other and know each other well. Most non-clinical and treatment discussion activity takes place in this zone.
Social distance	The range is 1-4 metres for people working in teams or groups such as in business and office. The zone within which the dental team operates.
Public distance	Beyond 4 metres. Eye-to-eye contact is limited and non-verbal feedback from facial gestures has little importance, as it cannot be perceived.

Anthropologist Edward Hall describes four categories of personal space (see Table 4-1). We must always beware of the intimacy of the area of space in which we engage with our patients. Our body orientation within this space sends important non-verbal signals to the patients. Lean towards them and it is a sign of interest; lean away and you indicate apathy and disinterest. In the intimate distance zone, we are ideally placed to read facial expressions. If you do not look at your patients, you will be perceived as indifferent, disinterested or even incompetent. Gaze aversion is a phenomenon that afflicts dentists when discussions take place about subjects that cause embarrassment – like fees – and this is likely to elicit a negative reaction from the patient. A lyric in Kenny Rogers' version of *The Gambler* reflects on a card player's ability to "read people's faces", which sums it all up rather neatly.

Observe the posture of your patients – anxiety leads to a tense and rigid posture. In contrast, a relaxed posture is a sign of comfort and confidence. By recognising these cues, you should then aim to deal with what you read into the posture. For example, a patient struggling in the dental chair may be indicative of lack of comfort. If you notice this and adjust the chair and perhaps reposition the headrest, it shows clearly that you are patient focused.

Where does all this fit into the business of dentistry? It is part of being patient-centred − you should have the ability to "read people's faces" without the need for vocalisation. Act on what you read, and you will have created a small but highly significant link in the service-profit chain.

The e-Revolution

Recent developments in computers, telecommunications and access to the Internet represent a convergence of technologies that is set to transform the way that the business of dentistry will operate in the future. A detailed discussion on the subject is beyond the scope of the present text but will be fully explored in another title in the series.

The e-revolution will force us all to rethink many of our traditional paradigms, and we need to consider exactly what implications this technological convergence will have on the business of dentistry. Unlike the other channels of communication, electronic communications lack emotion. It is a matter-of-fact medium existing as text on a screen often devoid of emotional content and lacking the human touch. Its applications will undoubtedly evolve, but in a people business, which is so heavily focused on care, the e-message is difficult to deliver with empathy. If you communicate via email with patients, remember that it is private correspondence between the sender and the recipient and is subject to the same code of confidentiality and disclosure as any paper record.

Websites

There is no doubt that patients are seeking credible and authoritative information on the Internet. If you are going to use your website for conveying this information, remember to make the content patient-friendly. The design and content must reflect an understanding of the patient's perception and level of understanding about dentistry. The design must be in empathy with the patient experience.

It is becoming increasingly important for websites to implement security and privacy standards, which reassure patients that their personal and transactional information will be kept confidential and secure.

A complete security solution has four elements:
1. Authentication (this identifies who the parties are).
2. Confidentiality (maintains the privacy of the communication).
3. Non-repudiation (makes the sent information irrevocable).
4. Integrity (ensures the contents are valid).

Use your website to convey information about your practice. Make advice sheets available for download and use the site to provide information about you, your practice and your team. The great advantage of the medium is the relatively low cost of updating information. With careful design and planning, you could do this yourself at minimal cost. Having a practice website sends a clear signal to your patients about your market position and, whilst the medium may lack the emotional value of face-to-face communications, it is an excellent for conveying information.

Regulation

In many respects the technology has overtaken the regulatory standards that serve to temper its application. At the time of writing, the American Accreditation Healthcare Commission is developing an accreditation programme for Internet healthcare sites. Its function will be to assist both healthcare workers and their patients to sort out the online "wheat from the chaff" in what is believed to be the first effort to create an accredited seal of approval for health sites. If the initiative is successful, it could help allay questions surrounding the reliability of the information on Internet health sites and how those sites protect their users' personal information. Standards covering candour, honesty, quality, informed consent, privacy, professionalism and accountability will be developed to reflect the growing use of the Internet.

Further Reading

Bewes T. Cynicism and Postmodernity. London: Verso, 1997.

Cherry C. On Human Communication. Cambridge: MIT Press, 1966.

Corah NL, O'Shea RM, Bissell GD, Thines TJ, Mendola P. The dentist–patient relationship: perceived dentist behaviors that reduce patient anxiety and increase satisfaction. J Am Dent Assoc 1988;116:73-76.

Dimbleby R, Burton G. More Than Words: An Introduction to Communication. London: Methuen, 1985.

Kulich KR. Interpersonal skills in the dentist–patient relationship. The art of dentistry. Doctoral dissertation (psychol.) Göteborg University, Sweden, 2000.

Marder E. The Laws of Choice. Predicting Customer Behavior. New York: The Free Press, 1997.

Chapter 5
Marketing

The Institute of marketing defines marketing as "the management process responsible for identifying, anticipating and satisfying customers' requirements profitably". Dun and Bradstreet claim that 48% of businesses fail because of *ineffective* marketing.

It is known that some dentists view the application of marketing techniques in their practice as an activity perilously close to breaching professional ethics. One major concern is that marketing involves "hard selling" and involves forms of "persuasion" and "coercion". This misinterpretation of the meaning of marketing is not restricted to the professions. Hugh Davidson, author and a visiting professor at Cranfield School of Management, writing in the magazine *Marketing*, expressed the view that the "m" word should be replaced because of its "deeply confusing double meaning". He argues that the word fails to distinguish between "the substance of marketing, and its abuse, which stems from its association with spin doctoring, manipulation and the flashier end of selling". His solution is to use the phrase "demand management". It may be that dentists uncomfortable with the "m" word will find its replacement more acceptable. Whatever the choice of phrase, the core principles of marketing remain and their effective application is essential for success in the business of dentistry.

There are a number of ways in which marketing principles can be applied successfully in the business of dentistry.

Word-of-mouth Marketing

In *Liberation Management*, Tom Peters describes word–of–mouth marketing as "the most powerful force in marketing". He writes that the statement is as true for Boeing as it is for The Body Shop, and the business of dentistry is no different.

Word of mouth marketing is the only promotional method that is of patients, by patients, and for patients. It is the quintessential sign of success. It works for the simple reason that the sender has nothing to gain from the receiver's subsequent actions; it has been determined that 70% of people rely on the advice of others when selecting their doctor or dentist.

It is inevitable that some people will be better positioned to recommend your services than others. They are sometimes referred to as network hubs – researchers like to call them "opinion leaders"; industry calls them "influencers". They are individuals who

- Have accurate information about your practice.
- Receive added value that they attend.
- Receive excellent service from you and your team.
- Are in a position where others may ask them for advice.
- Have direct experience of your responsiveness to their problems.
- Believe that you are able to exceed their positive expectations.
- Are proud to be associated with your practice.

From a marketing point of view, it is important to try and identify these individuals because they are key players in the grapevine that is word–of–mouth marketing.

Michael Cafferky's belief in word–of–mouth marketing is absolute. Author of *Patients Build Your Practice: Word-of-mouth Marketing for Healthcare Practitioners,* he makes some interesting observations about the concept:

- People like to talk. They talk because they feel.
- People like to talk about things of mutual interest.
- Some people get listened to more than others.
- Word-of-mouth communication is the primary means by which your reputation is spread.
- Word-of-mouth is regarded as the best method to signal value to patients.
- Word-of-mouth is controlled by your patients.
- Patients who spread your reputation can expand and exaggerate your virtues or faults when you cannot.
- The central figure in word-of-mouth communication is the "opinion leader". Cafferky suggests that 20–40% of the population are perceived as opinion leaders.
- Word of mouth covers the largest proportion of the population compared with any other promotional method.
- Negative word of mouth travels faster than positive word of mouth and helps potential patients to discriminate on one or more product/service attributes.

Internal Marketing

Internal marketing consists of those activities in your practice involving the existing patient base that enhance your image and set you apart as being uniquely attractive. Properly executed internal marketing lays the ground for effective word-of-mouth marketing. It compels your patients to tell their family members and friends about your unique and special practice. Here are some internal marketing ideas used in many practices that are said to deliver positive outcomes:

- Make follow-up telephone calls in the evening to each patient who has experienced a difficult procedure.
- Provide warm towels to start and/or finish each visit. (Clearly an idea borrowed from the airline industry.)
- Prepare a practice portfolio in the reception area containing letters of appreciation and "thank you" notes from your patients. (Ask their permission for inclusion first to avoid a breach in confidentiality.)
- Prepare a photo portfolio of clinical cases showing "before" and "after" images.
- Acknowledge special events in the lives of your patients by appropriate gestures of goodwill – cards or "gifts" which will remind them.
- Issue a welcome pack to all new patients.

External Marketing

External marketing includes the range of activities you undertake which are targeted to potential new patients outside your practice. It also includes a range of promotional initiatives that are discussed later in this chapter.

Marketing Strategy

The marketing strategy particularly relevant to the business of dentistry includes:

The SWOT analysis

Any organisation must have an understanding of its strengths and weakness and a sense of direction and purpose if it is survive in business. The business of dentistry is no exception. The practice image and its strengths and weaknesses must be carefully studied. Objective assessments can be made using the SWOT analysis, a tool for marketing audit. This analysis helps to identify the strengths and weaknesses of the practice and its team as well as pos-

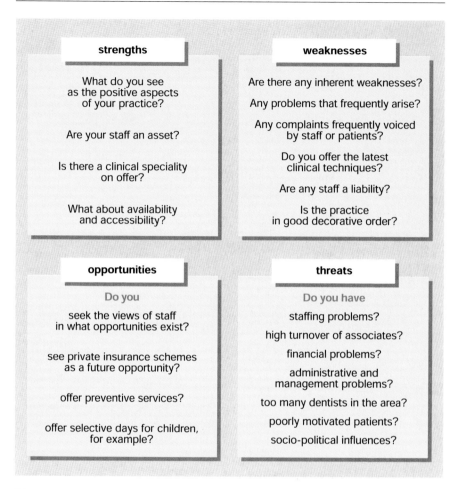

Fig 5-1 SWOT analysis.

sible opportunities and threats. A typical SWOT analysis should answer some key questions (see Fig 5-1).

When considering opportunities and threats, your analysis of the situation can be helped by trying to order your thoughts in a meaningful way. One way to do this is to use a matrix format (see Figs 5-2 and 5-3). The threat matrix is a reminder that we should not focus on concerns that fall into quadrant 4 – those that pose little threat and are unlikely to occur. In contrast,

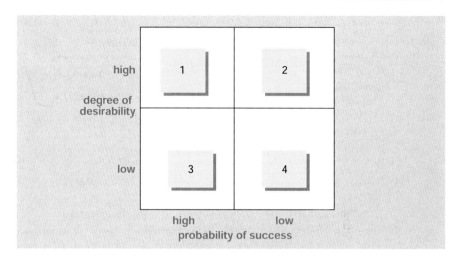

Fig 5-2 The opportunity matrix.

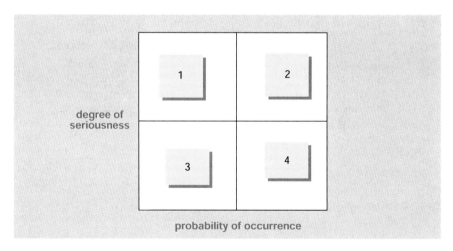

Fig 5-3 The threat matrix.

threats in quadrant 1 demand a strategic approach to include an element of contingency planning.

The PEST analysis
This is a tool for analysing the likely impact of environmental change on the organisation. PEST stands for:

- **P**olitical/legal
- **E**conomic/competitive
- **S**ocial/cultural
- **T**echnological.

The PEST analysis can be used to identify any factors under each of the four headings that may have an impact on your practice and the significance of those factors. For example, changes in government policy may affect the extent and nature of the range of treatments that may be available under, for example, the NHS.

Changes in the economic climate can have a direct impact on spending power amongst patients. The extent of the impact will vary from one part of the country to another and can also vary within a local community. The so-called "feel-good factor" amongst home owners when interest rates are low and house price inflation is high is one example of how the state of the economy affects the mood of consumers.

Social changes can also affect your practice. More women now go out to work and people are tending to work longer hours. This could have an affect on when your practice is open. It is known that couples are waiting longer before they start a family and in some areas the role of the extended family is greater than in others. For example, in one practice limited to orthodontics, the dentist made the observation that almost 30% of the private fee income for the practice was derived not from the parents of the children he treated, but the grandparents. Local factors can be very important and it is important to be aware of the social trends in your area.

Technology has made a huge impact on our lives and you should be aware what impact the age of information technology and the Internet will have on your practice. Does your practice reflect this modern age or do you need to invest to deliver the increase in expectations from your patients?

The marketing mix
The marketing mix concept is long established. It consists of a range of ingredients that can be blended to create a unique mix for your practice. The mix should be unique to the practice and its environment and help achieve your vision for your business. In other words, the ingredients should be blended to suit your objectives and priorities in much the same way as a chef blends ingredients to achieve the desired result. The ingredients of the marketing mix are shown in Fig 5-4.

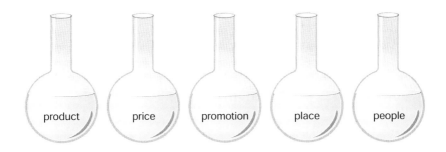

Fig 5-4 The ingredients of the marketing mix.

The product

The products and services offered by your practice should aim to satisfy patient needs. The quality of the products of dentistry (restorations, root canal treatments, for example) may not be always obvious to patients. The same is true of some clinical outcomes. For example, a patient may fail to recognise the quality of treatment where there has been resolution of an apical area following root canal treatment unless the patient has been equipped with the necessary information to make that judgement. What is tangible to the dentist may therefore be intangible to the patient. The patient will, however, demand elements of quality in the manner in which the treatment was provided.

The product in the business of dentistry comprises three elements. These are the product's attributes, its benefits and the service elements related to its delivery. They are shown in Fig 5-5.

The price

Clearly, the cost of dental care is an important factor in the business of dentistry. The issue is complex because the impact of price on a patient is related not only demographic variables but to complex issues like perception of value and spending priorities. The price-effect principles proposed by Eric Marder suggest that on average a price increase of 10% will produce a share decrease of around 9%, but there is a great variability in this result. One time in five the loss will be much larger, and one time in five there will be no loss at all. One reason for these inconsistent results may be perceptions of value and worth.

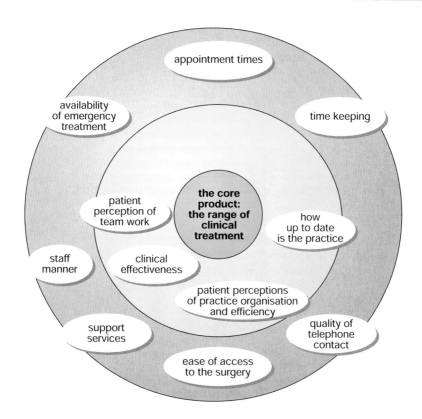

Fig 5-5 The three elements of the dental product.

Your market positioning will determine the perception of value amongst your patients. The budget airline industry has shown that the commercial marketplace is price sensitive and that a low price on what is seen as an acceptable level of service (in this case transportation) is clearly an advantage. An organisation that is customer focused is likely to have a service advantage over one that is not. The relationship of price and service quality advantages is illustrated in Fig 5-6.

Low-service quality but a high price advantage. This is the no frills option, like the budget airline model: a core service with a distinct price advantage. The practice offers a basic service which addresses the core need but must closely control business costs and relies on high volume throughput.

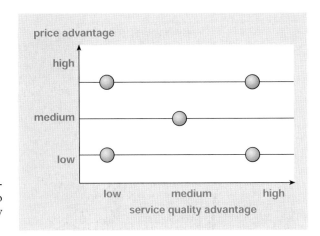

Fig 5-6 Market positioning in relation to price and service quality advantages.

High-service quality advantage but a low price advantage. The practice offers a high quality service at a premium price. It is positioned at the luxury end of the market. Margins are high to compensate for reduced market share. It reflects a high-quality private practice.

Medium-service quality advantage and a medium price advantage This is the middle ground. It reflects the status of the so-called "independent practice".

High-service quality advantage coupled with a high price advantage The model to strive for where patients receive exceptional service at a competitive price. Organisations who achieve this status are models of excellence. They are less expensive than their competitors but provide the same level of quality service.

It is worth remembering the Gucci family motto: "Quality is remembered long after the price is forgotten."

Promotion

Promotion is about communication. It is about finding ways of communicating benefits of products and services to patients in way that makes them appreciate quality and recognise value. Methods include advertising, interpersonal exchanges, paper-based communication and the Internet. The important thing to remember is that any type of practice promotion must adhere to the highest ethical standards:

- It must not contain any false, inaccurate, misleading, confusing, fraudulent, ambiguous or deceptive statements or claims.
- It must not create false or unjustified expectations of favourable results.

Table 5-1. **The "AIDA" test**

Attention	Does your advertisement grab the reader's attention? Look at the layout, design and choice of images in the advertisement.	✓
Interest	Having attracted attention, is the content of the advertisement interesting? How could you make it more interesting to the reader?	✓
Desire	Is the product or service you are advertising relevant to the market at which the advertisement is aimed? Will it create a desire for the product or service?	✓
Action	Does the advertisement inspire people to want to access your services? Remember that action can follow many months after the desire has been created. Don't be hasty and expect immediate results from your advertisement.	✓

- It must not, either by the nature or the manner or frequency of dissemination, be undignified, in bad taste, sensational or otherwise offensive.
- Any initiative that may be considered flamboyant, grandiose or sensational is best avoided because it may not be in the interest of the profession.

Advertising is a frequently used promotional activity. It has been described as little more than a game of chance, with most specialists in the field acknowledging that half of advertising does not work, although but no one quite knows *which* half. One useful way to approach your advertising initiative is to follow the acronym "AIDA" (Table 5-1), which describes and defines the process. For an advertisement to have the desired effect it must first attract "attention". It must be of "interest" to the reader, then it must create "desire" for the product or service it relates to, and inspire the reader towards "action". This four-step process is a useful planning tool in dental practice and any advertising initiative should pass the AIDA test

The message in your promotional material is made up of two components (Fig 5-7). Eric Marder puts forward a similar view in what he calls his "Law of Persistence". This states that "the effect produced by a message is made up of two components: a transient effect and an intrinsic effect. The transient effect decays rapidly. The intrinsic effect lasts indefinitely".

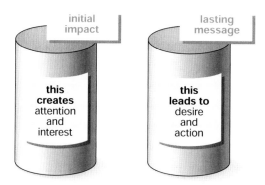

Fig 5-7 Promotional material made up of two components.

We should remember that consistency is important. Your existing and potential patients will look for consistency and congruence in your advertising material, in your environment and in the word-of-mouth messages they get from others, and they will relate this to their own experiences. A good advertisement cannot overcome deficiencies in service or product quality because when this consistency is lacking patients will rely on actual experience – their own or that of someone else.

Some practices apply the principles of "reminder advertising", which uses a range of advertising specialities that are given free of charge to your patients with your practice name, address and phone number on them. These could include ballpoint pens, calendars, advice sheets, mugs, etc. They can also be free samples of what you sell – like toothbrushes.

The Place

Access and environmental factors are important in this ingredient. The image of the practice, external and internal design cues and ambience play important parts in the marketing mix. The practice design and décor should reflect a professional and caring environment and will help to convert the intangible elements of service quality to the tangible benefits that can be seen in the physical environment. This conversion is about engaging the senses.

The People

In the business of dentistry, like in any other people business, we must

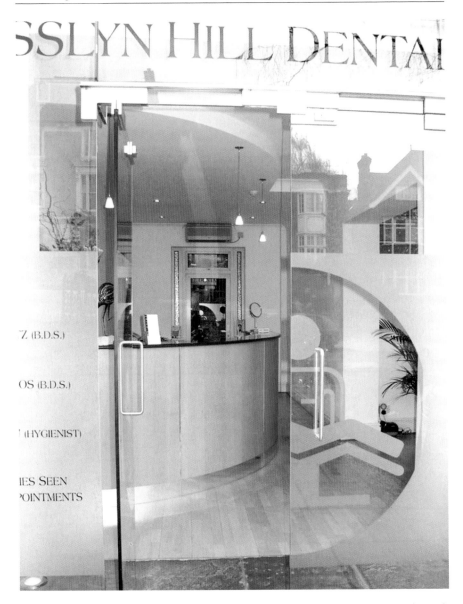

Plate 5-1. The exterior of a practice in a residential area. The combination of wood, metal and glass reflects the modern approach to dentistry.

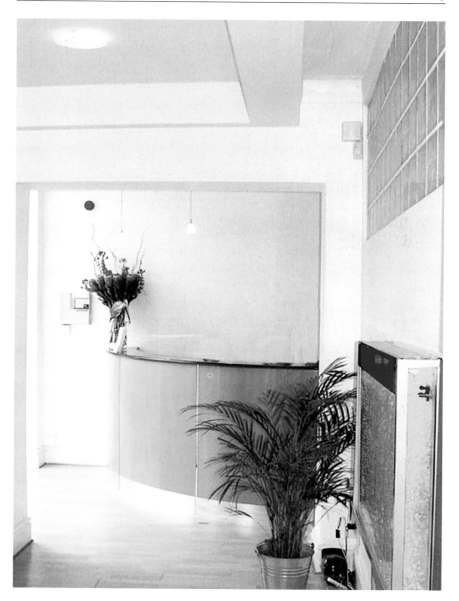

Plate 5-2. Internal view from a different angle. Note how the design incorporates the effect of natural light, which bathes the front desk through the glass doors shown in Plate 5-1.

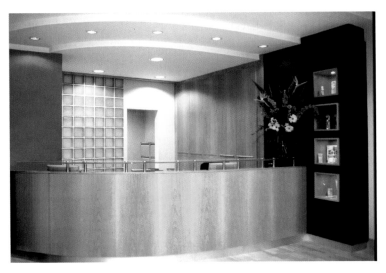

Plate 5-3. Reception area in a spacious environment in a practice sited in a busy retail area. Note the use of curves that is reflected in the ceiling design. The image is modern, reflected in the choice of materials.

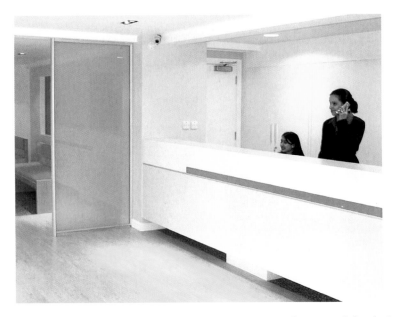

Plate 5-4. Linear reception area. There are no curved areas and the design is more angular.

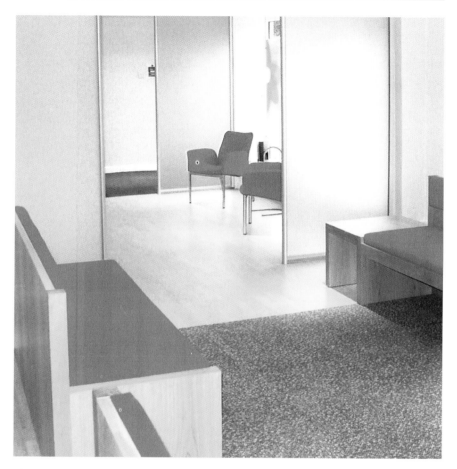

Plate 5-5. Angular, straight-lined theme continued in the choice of furnishings and in the design of floor areas and partitions.

remember that people buy people. The patients who travel for miles to return to their dentist do so because of trust and not the practice décor or the television in the ceiling. Those elements may have played a part in attracting those patients in the first place, but once the relationship has been established the human factor is dominant.

Your commitment to people begins with your commitment to your team. Their behaviour and actions will have an impact on patients' perceptions. Recruitment, training, motivation and reward are just some of the issues to

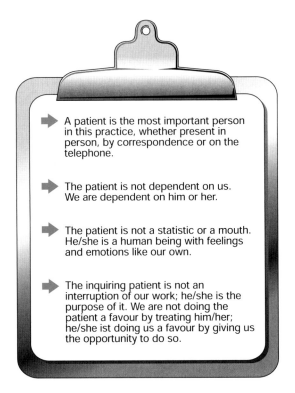

Fig 5-8 The patient (after Gordon Selfridge's memo to his staff defining a customer).

consider when building your winning team.

We have all heard and no doubt recited one of the mantras of business: "the customer comes first". Hal Rosenbluth, CEO of Rosenbluth Travel and co-author of *The Customer Comes Second*, admits that his secret of success is "controversial [because] it centres around [the] basic belief that companies must put their people – not their customers – first". Rosenbluth's view makes a lot of sense. He justifies his stance by suggesting, "When a company puts its people first, the results are spectacular. They are inspired to provide a level of service that truly comes from the heart. It cannot be faked." Adopting Rosenbluth's view, the focus of the team must be on the welfare of the patient. This is perhaps best summarised in the memo to his staff "defining a customer" from founder of the eponymous London department store, Gordon Selfridge, adapted to the dental practice as Fig 5-8.

Position

The term "positioning" is used to describe the reputation of a business in its community. It is very important to understand the distinction between image and reputation. Image is how you think you see yourself but reputation is how others perceive you. Positioning is about how you distinguish your practice from others in the marketplace. You can do this through:

Product features This is very common in industry but has limited application in dental practice unless your practice offers unique products or services. Examples include dental lasers, implants, CAD-CAM restorative options, or particular tooth-whitening techniques.

Benefits This follows on from product-based positioning but relies on talking to patients to inform them about what your product or service can do for them. The features on your CEREC machine may be state-of-the-art technology, but unless patients can be made to understand what the benefits will be to them, you may not capture the market. Remember patients buy benefits.

User category This can be a useful technique particularly when marketing cosmetic treatment options. When the treatment or procedure has been used or demonstrated by models with whom your patients can identify, an association is formed.

Positioning against a competing business Your approach could be an implicit or an explicit comparison but remember that it must remain ethical. The implicit approach is subtler, but explicit comparisons are more direct. It is a strategy that has been adopted by some dentists who make direct price comparisons – for example, with neighbouring competitors from the corporate sector.

Product class disassociation A less common type of positioning. It is particularly effective when used to introduce a new product that differs from traditional products. Mercury-free restorations are new product classes positioned against traditional dental amalgam.

G. Lynn Shostack, writing in 1987, suggested that positioning strategy should be based on "structural complexity and structural diversity". Complexity relates to the steps necessary to deliver the service and diversity relates to how variable the service output is. Diversity of outcomes is less likely in a smaller practice where it is easier to implement controls and consistency. A large practice may elect to downsize but retain its range of existing services that will then be provided by fewer clinicians, thereby reducing the likelihood of variations in clinical outcome.

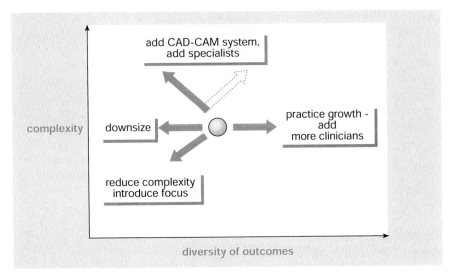

Fig 5-9 Shifting your market position.

A practice may choose to increase complexity – for example, by offering in-house specialist services, or introducing modern techniques like a CAD-CAM system. In this scenario, diversity could reduce if all specialists were working to the same service standards (see Fig 5-9). Indeed, this happens in the dental corporate sector where specialists are contracted to work for the same group but in different sites. If, however, individuals work in environments that set different service standards then scope for diversity increases (shown in Fig 5-9 by the dotted line). The same can be said of clinicians who work with the CAD-CAM system, for example. If they are all equally well trained and experienced diversity is low, but it could be high if their relative competence with the system is markedly different.

Diversity of outcomes can compromise the image of the practice. It has been suggested that low diversity and low complexity environments operate more effectively and operate in so-called niche markets. Heskett has concluded that businesses achieve high profitability by having either market focus or operating focus. He concludes, "organisations that achieve both market and operating focus are nearly unbeatable".

From a clinical point of view, diversity of outcomes can be likened to variance in the concept of the clinical pathway, where consistency is seen as an important benefit of a given pathway.

Market Segmentation

Segmentation is a technique of dividing the market into smaller discrete slices and targeting each with a modified or specific product or service. It is known that markets and customers who form those markets are fluid. The "market" is not static; it is a dynamic interaction of social groups. These individual groups are segments of the whole. No consumer market is static; few segments are the same today as, say, ten years ago.

Without targeted efforts, a vast proportion of marketing and public relations effort is a waste of valuable resources. There are a number of segment classifications that can help in practice development. Instead of marketing a product in just one way to everyone, we should recognise that some segments are not only different, but better (better meaning more receptive) than others for a particular product or service. This approach can be helpful in penetrating markets that would otherwise be too broad and undefined without segmentation. Markets are often segmented using demographic and psychographic variables. Demographics is the study of the distribution, density and vital statistics of a population, and includes such characteristics as:

- sex
- age
- education
- geographic location
- home ownership (against renting)
- marital status
- size of family unit
- total income of family unit
- ethnic or religious backgrounds
- job classification (blue collar versus salaried or professional).

Psychographics is the study of how the human characteristics of consumers may have a bearing on their response to products, packaging, advertising and marketing efforts. Behaviour may be observed and is influenced by:

Predisposition What is there about a person's past culture, heredity or upbringing that may influence their perception of dental health or attitude to dentistry?

Influences What parts do education and peer pressure play in determining a patient's acceptance of a treatment plan or their attendance pattern?

Product attributes What the product is or can be made to represent in the minds of consumers can have a significant bearing on whether certain market segments will accept it. These attributes can be communicated through marketing efforts.

The areas to look at and the questions to consider are summarised in Table 5-2.

Table 5-2. **The message in your promotional material**

Price/value perception	Is the item worth the price being asked?
Quality	What can be said about the quality of the materials?
Benefits	How does the patient feel after receiving the product?
Trust	Can the patient rely on your brand? What about the reputation of the provider of the product, i.e. the dentist and/or the practice?

Table 5-3. **The 7-step marketing plan**

1. Define your pur— pose and have a clear vision of what you want to achieve.	In order to create a truly successful marketing plan, you must decide what it is you want to accomplish and then picture it already being a success. Remember Covey's "All things are created twice" habit. Assemble a team of others who share the same vision of success. Together, create a well-defined marketing plan. The objective is to communicate quality service and quality care to patients while simultaneously taking care of your team and yourself.
2. Think about your strategy	Make sure the strategies have clear and specific expectations of performance for everyone involved. Put your plan in writing - starting with the end result - working back to the initial starting-point. Use the principles discussed in this chapter about positioning and segmentation.
3. Be prepared to invest in your vision	Investment is not just about money: it is about time and energy. Spend time thinking about what you want to do and how you will do it. Take the time to discuss strategy with others and to look in the general market place to see how other service organisations approach similar challenges.

4. Implement the plan	Collate all the information you have gathered so far and put it into action. Be consistent in your actions. Remember to involve the dental team and to ensure that each team member is aware of and accountable for his or her part of the plan.
5. Gather feedback	Remember that one of Carl Sewell's strategies for keeping customers for life is to measure everything – so measure outcomes constantly, daily, weekly, monthly, quarterly. Different initiatives will give results in a different timeframe. Be prepared to wait for results but also be prepared to make changes and modifications based on feedback. Use feedback and close the loop. Don't forget to seek views from your team – remember your team is a valuable resource.
6. Leadership	Effective leadership is the key ingredient to keeping the plan on course. Be positive, diverse, enthusiastic and, above all, inspirational.
7. Repeat the process	Remember that marketing is an ongoing activity. The market is changing all the time. Repeat and revise your strategy to stay in touch with today's marketplace. Don't take the risk of standing still.

The Marketing Plan

A good marketing plan is essential if your practice is to meet the combined challenges of change and competition. It should be a guide on which you will base decisions and should ensure that every member of the practice team is working together to achieve the same goals. The marketing plan must take into consideration your vision for the practice and must be closely aligned to the business plan.

Before your marketing plan can be developed, ask yourself:
For whom are you designing your services (market segmentation)?
What should that service mean to those in the marketplace (market positioning)?
The 7-step guide in Table 5-3 will help you to develop a marketing plan to support your strategy. Your marketing strategy provides the "how" and the direction for the course of action. With your strategy in place, you must now focus on the tactical aspects and it is from this that the timelines, resources and budget considerations for the marketing plan are derived.

Further Reading

Cafferky ME. Patients Build Your Practice: Word-of-mouth Marketing for Health-care Practitioners. New York: McGraw-Hill Publishing, 1994.

Heskett JL, Sasser WE, Schlesinger LA. The Service Profit Chain: How Leading Companies Link Profit and Growth to Loyalty, Satisfaction, and Value. New York: The Free Press, 1997.

Rosenbluth HF. The Customer Comes Second and Other Secrets of Exceptional Service. New York: William Morrow and Company, 1992.

Shostack GL. Service positioning through structural change. J Market 1987;51: 34–43.

Chapter 6
The Basic Principles of Finance

All businesses, however large or small, require finance and as long as the business continues to trade this will always be the case. It is important to understand that all privately owned dental practices are businesses and, therefore, require to be financed. If the practice is the body, then finance is the blood supply and a healthy practice requires a healthy and balanced blood supply. Dental practices are financed from two sources: owners' capital combined with an external source.

Owners' Capital

The owners of all dental practices finance the business, either in whole or in part. If there is no external borrowing, then that particular practice will be fully funded by its owners. The owners' capital is normally a combination of monies originally put in to start or take over the individual practice, together with retained earnings (profits generated year on year but not drawn from the business). A well-run practice should show an increased retained capital investment from its owners.

One important aspect that is often overlooked is that the retained capital within the business should earn a better rate of return from the profits of the practice than would be obtained by placing those monies on deposit or in to an alternative investment elsewhere. This nature of return is known as the Internal Rate of Return (IRoR) and it is an important financial ratio. If the owner can achieve 5% on monies invested externally, then the IRoR should be in excess of this figure.

External Finance

There are numerous ways in which a practice owner can finance the purchase or development of the individual practice, utilising outside money. In the vast majority of cases, practices are financed to some extent by external borrowing. If your borrowing is appropriately structured and for a specific purchase, it means that you are able to develop your individual business much faster than would be the case relying on your own finance resources. It is very important to bear in mind that all debt has ultimately to be repaid, together with the relevant interest, which is the reward to the external lender.

Borrowing Money

There are some golden rules when it comes to borrowing money for your practice.

1. Minimise non tax-deductible borrowing

In the vast majority of cases, domestic mortgage borrowing does not enjoy any tax relief whatsoever, since the demise of MIRAS. It is therefore essential to review all domestic mortgage loans on a regular basis: lump sum or enhanced monthly payments can make a dramatic difference to the term of the mortgage.

2. Ensure that the term of the finance arrangement is shorter than the life of the asset

As an example, it is self-defeating to finance computers or similar investment over periods of more than three years, as the depreciation rates of such equipment are extraordinarily high.

3. Do not be afraid to structure certain borrowings on a secured basis, if it provides a substantially better interest rate

It is understandable for an individual to be reticent to offer a Charge on their domestic or other property in favour of the lender. However, it should be understood that if money is borrowed lenders will always seek full repayment at the appropriate time – whether the loan is secured or not.

4. Take professional advice when signing any new agreement

Comparing APRs can often be very difficult and the devil can be in the detail. Ensure that you fully understand the commitment that you are entering into, particularly if there are any secondary periods or balloon rentals involved (a balloon rental is a deferred payment at the end of a finance lease, lease purchase, contract purchase or personal contract purchase).

5. Regularly review all finance arrangements

This is more essential now than ever before as the market becomes increasingly competitive. There is no law against talking with your lenders from time to time to ensure that you are still enjoying the most competitive products.

6. Repay all debt as soon as possible
Even if a loan is tax deductible, that does not mean it should not be repaid
if surplus funds are available. If you enjoy tax relief at 40% this means that
the remaining 60% of the interest charge is still financed by you and the cash
flow burden of the loan repayments remains. It is therefore essential that all
long-term loan commitments allow for early repayment of part or the entire
loan without penalty.

Having established the rules, let us consider the different types of financing
that are appropriate to modern dental practice.

Freehold Property

In general terms, freehold property assets have an extremely long life and
therefore can be financed over a long period of time – typically 20–25 years.
The financing of such assets through individual pension arrangements has
become increasingly popular over the last few years and can have significant
tax benefits. However, personal circumstances will often dictate as to the
best structure for such borrowings.

Fixed rates of interest on loans to buy property can be extremely advanta-
geous and are normally arranged on a five- or ten-year basis by most of the
main clearing banks. The right answer, of course, requires a very clear crys-
tal ball, but fixing rates when the base rate is low can often be seen to be very
sensible and years later, when rates have moved up again, you will have the
satisfaction of still paying at the lower fixed rate. Such arrangements also have
the benefit of allowing for accurate budgeting of your financial overheads
over a reasonable period of time.

In certain circumstances it is quite acceptable to secure the lending required
for the practice property – and indeed other assets, if appropriate – on the
proprietors' domestic residences if this provides a lower rate of interest, but
once again professional advice is essential.

Dental Equipment

Good-quality equipment if well maintained should last at least ten years. Statistics indicate that on average dental surgeries in the UK are refurbished
every fourteen years; many, of course, stay as they are for much longer. Practitioners do not appear to appreciate the benefits of regular re-equipping (a
seven-year cycle would not be unreasonable) in terms of operating efficiency

and modern presentation to your patient base. It is understood that new surgery investment (of the right quality) is not cheap, but there should be no difficulty in amortising the costs over a seven-year period. In fact, the vast majority of individual surgery investments are financed over a five-year term, either on a bank loan, lease purchase or finance lease arrangement.

Leasing

The tax treatment of the finance lease is very different from that of the loan or lease purchase arrangement, in that the equipment is rented for a primary period and the rentals are charged against the trading income of the practice each year. If the lease is therefore for a primary period of five years, tax relief is given equally over this initial period. At the end of this primary term there is normally a peppercorn secondary rental paid to the finance house and the equipment is not normally ever owned by the practice (although you have the full benefit of the equipment financed in this way).

The bank loan or lease purchase agreement provides for an initial allowance of 40% of the cost (under current legislation) and then a depreciating allowance over the succeeding years. Under this arrangement the total allowances received over the five years of the finance agreement are 81% of the total cost of the investment, but the investor has received the benefit of a relatively high initial element of tax relief in year one.

If the practitioners' cash flow is strong, then a very attractive alternative is a three-year finance lease, which ensures that one-third of the tax relief is enjoyed in each of the three years following the investment. Apart from the peppercorn rental in the secondary period, referred to above, the total cost of the investment is therefore written off against tax on a straight-line basis over this three-year term. The market for equipment finance is extremely competitive and therefore it certainly pays to shop around.

Second-hand Equipment

It should be noted that a pure finance lease should never be used for second-hand equipment; this will attract an unnecessary charge to VAT.

Goodwill

Purchasing goodwill can be an extremely worthwhile investment and should have a significant life. Most Lenders, however, will not wish to lend on goodwill over such a long period as with freehold property. The normal term of such loans is ten years, but up to fifteen years can be considered. As is the case with second-hand dental equipment, finance leases are definitely not an appropriate product for financing the purchase of goodwill.

IT Equipment

Under current Inland Revenue rules, dental practices can purchase new computer (and similar) equipment and enjoy 100% tax relief immediately. In general, therefore this means that a finance lease is totally inappropriate for such investment as it will unnecessarily spread the tax relief beyond year one.

Most practices will still need to spread the monthly payments and this is easily achieved by way of a three-year bank loan or lease purchase structure. It is essential that the financing arrangements for computer and similar equipment are for short periods only as such assets depreciate faster than ice cream in the Sahara Desert and quality practices will need to reinvest in IT, in accord with this three-year cycle.

Working Capital

All practices have cash flow variations throughout the trading cycle and some of these can be very substantial. Without doubt the best form of finance for working capital is an overdraft with a clearing bank and, once again, the rates of interest offered to good practices are now extremely competitive.

Overdraft borrowing is a cheap form of finance. The bank account is receiving money on a continuous basis, which effectively depresses the overdrawn balance, and the overdraft interest is calculated on the individual daily balance. It can be appreciated therefore that substantial bankings (e.g. monies from the Dental Practice Board and/or monthly credits from capitation schemes or individual patient payments in cases of extensive treatment plans) can have a significant impact on the overall interest charges on such an account.

On occasion, practices make substantial tangible asset investment out of an overdraft and then realise that a "hard core" element has built up within the balance. When this happens it can be useful to discuss with the bank the possibility of removing the hard-core element on to a separate loan to be repaid over a suitable period.

In general terms, these are the protocols for financing modern dental practices. As indicated, you should always dialogue with your accountant or business consultant to ensure the right structure for the financing that you require. Sensible financial planning certainly pays dividends in terms of cash flow management and maximisation of profit.

Financial Management of the Practice

It is essential for all practice owners to take responsibility for the financial management of their practice positively and proactively. In this regard, proper financial accounting systems are very important.

Cash Flow

As indicated previously, a healthy practice requires proper financing and the day-to-day financial requirements of each practice are provided by income from the patients. All team members should, therefore, understand that there is an average requirement of income to the practice each day and this should be published internally and monitored.

Clearly there will be variations on a day-to-day basis and particularly large elements of income will be received, either from completion of large treatment plans, NHS schedule payments or capitation scheme providers. Assuming that there is an overdraft facility in place (or excess funds on the practice bank account), variations in cash flow on a daily or weekly basis will be covered by movements within the bank account. However, falling cash balances or rising overdrafts over time provide the earliest indication of financial difficulties within a practice.

If your practice is short of cash flow, it can be tempting to restrict payments to suppliers (e.g. for materials and laboratory charges) to keep an overdraft facility within its limit. Such action may well please your bank manager temporarily, but unless you have an agreement to reduce payments to your key suppliers this may cause operational difficulties for the practice later on.

It should also be noted that the Inland Revenue are now much less tolerant of late payment of PAYE/NIC liabilities and therefore this form of secondary banking (i.e. building excess credit with the Revenue) is less likely than used to be the case. The Revenue have increased powers for charging interest on late-paid tax and interest charged by the Inland Revenue is never tax deductible.

Continuous monitoring of your cash flow is the simplest form of financial management and certainly the easiest to understand. The practice bank account receives money from the clinical activity of the practice, but pays money out in terms of direct costs, overheads, rewards to the team and personal drawings for the practice owner. Responsibility must therefore be taken by either the owner of the practice or, better still, the practice manager, to ensure the cash flow into the practice is maximised, so that debts are paid at the right time as they fall due (i.e. neither before nor after the due date of payment).

The basic principles of maximising cash flow in to the practice are:

1. Obtain part or full payment from each individual patient as early as possible in the treatment cycle.
2. Ensure that the practice can collect monies electronically, i.e. by Switch/Delta cards or credit cards. Electronic banking ensures minimal bad debts, speedy deposit of monies in to the practice bank account and, often, lower charges than clearing cheques. There is a great deal of competition amongst the banks in the provision of electronic banking to their customers and therefore the monthly costs are extremely low.
3. It there is any NHS activity within the practice all payment claim forms and requests for prior approval should be transmitted to the relevant payment Board by EDI link. It is therefore essential that such practices have an approved IT administration system to allow such transmissions to take place.
4. The utilisation of a discount – typically 5% – as an incentive to individual patients to pay for large treatment plans in toto at the commencement of treatment.

In terms of payments out of the practice bank account, all purchase invoices need to be logged as they come in and the due date for payment noted. It then becomes easier to forecast when these bills require to be paid and the impact on the practice cash flow at that time.

Break Even

In order properly to monitor practice cash flow it is important to understand the concept of "break even". All businesses have two types of cost: fixed and variable.

Fixed costs
These are the elements of overhead that do not change – or change only slightly – depending on the activity of the practice.

Such costs typically are:
- rent
- rates
- insurance
- light and heat
- telephone
- postage and stationery
- bank loans
- hire purchase and leasing payments
- professional fees
- personnel costs (wages and benefits)
- personal drawings.

Variable costs
The normal variable costs for most dental practice extend to:
- materials
- laboratory fees
- hygienist payments
- personnel costs (overtime or bonus payments).

These costs are variable as they move in line with the activity of the practice, i.e. the amount of work done. It should be noted that personnel costs that move in line with activity – particularly overtime for additional sessions worked – are regarded as variable costs.

A typical break-even graph is shown in Fig 6-1, indicating how practice profitability increases substantially the further away from the break-even point. Line F indicates the fixed cost element, and line V shows how variable costs rise with increased output. Line OR is the revenue line and its point of intersection with OV represents the break-even point for the business.

The business objective is to achieve the highest possible activity level beyond the break-even point. It is therefore extremely useful to recalculate the break-even point of a particular practice each trading year and then arrive at a new daily revenue collection target for immediate monitoring of the performance of the practice.

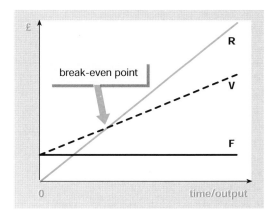

Fig 6-1 Typical break-even chart.

Dealing with Banks and Professional Advisers

It must be understood that these relationships with banks and professional advisers are extremely important, both for the practice itself and for the practice owner. The banking market for dental professionals in the UK is now more competitive than ever before. Good business propositions will be very attractive to the major lenders in the marketplace and it certainly pays to dialogue with two or three banks to find a combination of the best business offer and the right personal relationship. Two of the major clearing banks have now set up dedicated healthcare managers across the UK and it is their purpose to help dentists (and other medical practitioners) to achieve their business goals.

In dealing with the banks it is important to have the full support of your accountant or business adviser, so that both of you are fully confident in terms of what you want to achieve and what you require from your bank. The banks terms and conditions in respect of loan or overdraft monies should be transparent and specific for a certain period. It should also be clear that additional charges or tariffs will be applied to your account and in this respect it is perfectly proper to enquire of your bank how they can help you reduce the costs of running your facilities with them. In respect of your professional advisers: again, it is essential to have clear terms and conditions and you must fully understand what services are being provided to you and at what cost.

Outsourcing
Outsourcing of key activities can be an extremely effective way of minimising non-clinical pressure on your practice and can extend to:

- payroll
- human resources (contracts, job descriptions and appraisal systems)
- bookkeeping
- management accounts
- health and safety assessments
- clinical governance
- direct debit services for patient membership schemes, etc.

It is useful to review the activities within the practice that could be out-sourced, thus providing more time and energy for developing the practice internally.

Business Planning

Every business, including every dental practice, should have a business plan, which is written down. A written business plan is a combination of words and figures. The words describe the objective and the strategy for achieving the stated goals. The figures represent a forecast of cash flow, profits, and possible balance sheets in future years and provide an illustration of the likely financial outcome given the assumptions made.

It is important that the business plan provides a challenge, but is not overoptimistic. There is little worse than writing a two-year business plan and reaching the end of the first year to discover a significant shortfall compared to the forecast. This is demotivating. It also normally means a substantial revision of second-year forecasts and a new forecast for year three.

A sensible and professionally prepared business plan will achieve the right level of funding at the right price that is required and will normally include:
- future clinical activity
- team structure and training requirements
- marketing
- detailed financial projections (cash flows and projected profit-and-loss accounts)
- funding requirements of the practice.

Even if the reality is a much greater success than originally forecast, the plan should still be revisited to review the assumptions made and to assist the writing of a new plan for the next stage of development of the practice.

Tax Matters

Individual taxpayers are not under any obligation to maximise the amount of tax that is paid to the Inland Revenue. Having said that, it should also be understood that the Revenue are under strict control and direction from the Treasury to maximise the total tax take from the whole of the UK economy. It is therefore essential to take professional advice on a continuous basis in terms of profits being generated, new investment required and the tax status of certain team members (e.g. hygienists, dental assistants and associates). Tax legislation is becoming ever more complicated. The introduction of self-assessment in 1996/97 has given the Revenue greater powers and ensured that the burden of compliance has moved firmly on to the individual taxpayer and his or her agent.

All taxpayers must therefore ensure that apart from proper record keeping all their tax and financial affairs are kept completely up to date and in very good order. The objective must be to run your practice with a view to profit, but ensuring that at the same time the tax burden is kept under control. You should therefore take good professional advice legitimately to minimise the tax burden, thus preserving more of you own financial resources for reinvestment and further reward.

Chapter 7
Fee-setting

Many dentists have commented that the NHS fee scale is unable to deliver a realistic level of income to sustain all the costs of modern practice and provide the desired level of income to the individual practice owner. One of the most challenging, but ultimately satisfying aspects of private practice is the ability to set and revise your own fee scale independently of any third-party payment system. As soon as you deliver any element of care outside a fixed-fee third-party payment system (such as the NHS) you will have to, in some way shape or form, calculate the cost of that particular procedure and charge the patient accordingly.

Taking control of your fee setting is one true benefit of a successful move to private dentistry and allows an increasing number of practitioners to gain satisfaction and contentment beyond mere financial reward. However, financial success is essential to ensure the long-term stability and continued development of your practice. If insufficient income is generated, then even with strict cost control, the ability to sustain your practice over the longer term is not guaranteed.

There has been a tendency in the past for individual dentists to rely on a fee structure recommended by a particular professional group or body. This approach is inconsistent within the context of the business and is a flawed approach to fee setting. To use someone else's figures in respect of setting your own fees may prove to be a fundamental and expensive mistake and the philosophy of setting your own fees should be clear to all.

Method

One of the most important aspects is for each individual clearly to determine their future lifestyle. The allocation of time between work and relaxation is a relatively straightforward exercise but increasingly successful practitioners have been able legitimately to minimise their clinical commitment to a realistic level, whilst at the same time improving the quality of their social and family time. The major benefit of such an approach is clearly less stress and improved quality of life for the practitioner and their family.

The Variables

It is therefore very important that you are fundamentally honest in respect of:
- the number of clinical hours per week on a realistic basis
- the number of working weeks per year to allow for holidays and post-graduate development
- loss of chargeable time because it is impossible to achieve 100% efficiency.
- an accurate forecast of the total overheads structure of the practice based on fact and allowing for inflation and further investment
- a complete and comprehensive schedule of personal drawings, including forecast tax liability and realistic investment for retirement.

You must establish the facts of *your* practice and not simply take someone else's figures when analysing your cost base and income requirements. You must make a candid projection with regard to future operating costs. Inflation may be at an extremely low level, but experience suggests that dental practice inflation does not follow the Retail Price Index and operational changes in your practice may have significant impact on your cost base.

Schedule 1 (Table 7-1) shows details of the overall operating costs and income requirements for a single-handed principal already operating within the private sector. The personal drawings requirement of, say, £100,000 has been

Table 7-1. **Schedule 1: Operating costs 2003**

Payroll costs		£46,000
General overheads		£24,000
Financial costs		£18,000
Depreciation and amortisation		£12,000
Personal drawings		£100,000
	Total	£200,000
Add: Materials @ 7%		£14,000
Total income required excluding laboratory fees		**£214,000**

carefully scheduled to allow for all required expenditure, including the current tax provision based on the previous year's profits and increased pension investment (which is a factor and must never be ignored).

Once the overall costs of the practice, including drawings, have been determined, then it is important to calculate the available time as per Schedule 2 (Table 7-2). This makes the following assumptions:

- An average clinical (i.e. chairside) time of 32 hours per week.
- A normal working year of 46 weeks, allowing for statutory holidays, annual leave from the practice and a realistic level of postgraduate course attendance.
- The average downtime/non chargeable time is assumed to be 20%. If the downtime is more than 20%, then the practice has a problem, but a 20% discount of available clinical time should normally be conservative and should allow some latitude for the individual practitioner.

Table 7-2. **Schedule 2: Calculation of available hours**

9:00 am to 5:00 pm x 4 days =	28 hours
9:00 am to 1:00 pm x 1 day =	4 hours
Normal working week =	32 hours

32 hours per week x 46 weeks x 80% efficiency = 1,178 hours per annum

It can thus be determined that for this individual practice principal there should be at least 1,178 chargeable hours per annum. The sample practice also has a hygienist who works 4 days per week, and this should have a positive impact on the hourly rate required.

Initial Calculation

Schedule 3 (Table 7-3) details the calculation in this case, showing that the hygienist surgery makes a net contribution to overheads of £50,100 per annum. In the case of this particular practice, this allows for a reduction of up to £42.50 per hour in the target charge-out rate of the dentist's surgery. This is a reduction of 21% on the charge-out rate required, which is significant percentage.

All those who engage in the business of dentistry should undertake this basic

Table 7-3. **Schedule 3: Calculation of hourly rate**

Defined as

Annual total costs ÷ non-chargeable hours per annum = hourly rate

$$£215,000 ÷ 1,178 \text{ hours} = £182.50 \text{ per hour}$$

The use of hygienists for 4 days per week could reduce the hourly rate requirement for the dentist by £42.50 per hour, assuming:

1. 28 hours per week x 46 weeks x 80% efficiency = 1,030 hours per annum
2. 1,030 hours @ £80 per hour = increased income of £82,400
3. 1,888 paid hours @ £25 per hour = hygienist pay of £32,300

calculation. The calculations are a fundamental requirement in the financial management of the business.

It is at this stage that individual practitioners should carefully time all their clinical procedures and these timings should be on a realistic basis. It is particularly important that you calculate the time required to carry out a clinical procedure to a high standard and also include an allowance for patient communication – giving clinical advice and obtaining informed consent. There is absolutely no point in fudging this issue. It is tantamount to negligence to do so.

The mix of your patient base will also play an important part in the planning process. Some patient groups are low yield compared to others, and you will need to consider how to introduce compensatory mechanisms that allow you to maintain the average hourly targets set for your business.

Value Pricing

Increasingly, many practitioners find that the application of their standard hourly rate to the time requirement of an initial consultation or at a review examination can give rise to a suggested charge higher than they would wish. In such circumstances it is perfectly acceptable to allow for a reduced level of hourly income, particularly if such shortfall can be made up elsewhere.

In practice, the most common areas for making up this shortfall are items carrying laboratory costs (e.g. crowns, bridges, implants and dentures). Apart from laboratory-based work, periodontology, endodontics and orthodontics are also areas that can reasonably provide a much higher level of average hourly surgery income.

Once your fees have been set, resist the temptation continually to alter or amend them. An annual review should suffice unless there has been gross miscalculation of expenses. When the fees are due to be reset consider very carefully about possible changes in the overhead structure of the practice (particularly pay rates) and do not overlook forthcoming capital expenditure which is going to have a significant impact on the predicted overhead.

Comparisons

As indicated previously, utilising an average or adopted fee scale is not the route to financial success, but it should not be forgotten that your patients can compare. If at all possible it is important to verify your proposed fee scale with what else is being charged in the local marketplace – sometimes you may find that your charges are significantly lower than the other practices in the locality. In such cases, it might be useful to recalculate your figures, as forgetting to include your personal drawings requirement does have a fairly significant impact on your hourly rate!

Relatively small differences in fees between your own and other comparable practices do not normally cause a problem. However, if your charges are substantially higher than others in the area then further consideration may be required. On the other hand, it is not necessarily a major advantage if your charges are substantially lower than your local colleagues, as you may then end up attracting less-motivated and less-appreciative patients.

Publication

Every single member of staff should clearly understand the calculations and assumptions behind the hourly rate requirement. So it is a good idea to publish the fee guide and to refer to it when calculating treatment costs – to prevent what has been idiomatically become known as "oral-fiscal drag". The process goes something like this:

1. The dental brain calculates a charge of £450 for the work required.
2. The dental mouth (linked to some extent to the dental brain) delivers a quotation of £290 to the expectant and appreciative patient.
3. The delighted patient confirms acceptance with the response, "Is that all?"

4. The dental ear then conveys to the dental brain delight at non-rejection but misery at the dramatically negative impact on profitability!

Discounting your fees by 35% may indeed lessen the fear of rejection, but does not guarantee the creation of a sustainable practice.

One way of avoiding this common complaint is the utilisation of quality dental practice software, which allows the easy delivery of a fully detailed treatment plan properly costed and scheduled for consideration by the patient.

As well as computer systems, it is becoming increasingly common for individual practices to employ patient or treatment co-ordinators whose job is to discuss the cost of benefits arising from individual treatment plans and therefore the danger of a dentist under-pricing the treatment quotation is reduced. Successful medical practitioners have known for many years that discussion of fees is best left to others within their practices or consulting rooms.

Capitation

The major capitation providers are very willing to assist practitioners in terms of setting the different bands of monthly payments by individual patients. Such calculations must be scrutinised very carefully to ensure that all the figures are based on fact, with realistic assumptions. Practice owners must understand the impact of the cost of insurance administration, normally deducted from each monthly direct debit.

Two factors must be taken into account when considering capitation schemes. A patient's oral health condition varies over time and therefore regular recategorisation of patients amongst the fee bands is essential to ensure that the practice is neither under- nor overpaid for the care provided. Under normal capitation arrangements, it is the dentist who underwrites completely the oral health condition of the individual patient.

Membership Schemes

An increasingly popular alternative to pure capitation is that provided by a membership or access scheme. In this situation the individual patient pays the practice (normally via a third-party administrator) either monthly or quarterly for:

- Access to their preferred dentist for a specific number of examinations per annum.
- Attendance for hygienist treatment (similarly, for a specified number of visits per annum).
- Treatment at a discounted rate from the normal fee scale, as and when required.

Under such schemes it is normal for the individual patient to elect to pay an additional premium for trauma and accident cover and, therefore, under such a scheme this cost is not borne by the practitioner.

The advantage of such an arrangement can also be that there is likely to be an improved dialogue between dentist and patient in terms of working together to maintain oral hygiene. The individual patient also has more of a financial incentive in ensuring prevention of problems within their own mouth.

Summary

Irrespective of the particular arrangements in the individual practices, it should be appreciated that great care is required in terms of fee-setting calculations and the regular revision thereof.

In terms of planning a practice for profit, time spent on achieving the optimum level of fees is often much more productive than being over-concerned about cost reductions. Regular and realistic revision is a must and will ensure that the individual practice delivers a proper level of return on a continuous basis. At the same time this will ensure the value of the practice is maintained, thus allowing a very satisfactory disposal as and when required.

Chapter 8
Understanding Your Accounts

It is important to have an understanding of your accounts to monitor the financial status and success of your practice. These provide useful management information and can help to provide some guidance on developing the practice. A sample set of accounts is shown in Appendix 1 and should be referred to when reading this chapter.

Financial Statements

The most important financial statements are the balance sheet and the profit and loss account. A balance sheet is nothing more than a list of the assets accumulated and liabilities owed by the business. The difference between the two represents the net worth of the business. It provides a picture of the financial health of a business at a given moment, usually at the close of an accounting period. It lists a summary of the assets of the business, normally split between fixed and current assets, a summary of the liabilities of the business, and a summary of the owner's equity (the money owed to the owner of the business). The profit and loss account is an analysis of the performance of the business over the trading year, detailing what income was received, and what expenses were incurred.

The Balance Sheet

The balance sheet is designed to show how the assets, liabilities and net worth of a business are distributed at any given time. It can be prepared at regular intervals – for example, at each month's end, but especially at the end of each fiscal (accounting) year. By regularly preparing this summary of what the business owns and owes, the business owner or manager can identify and analyse trends in the financial strength of the business. It permits timely modifications, such as gradually decreasing the amount of money the business owes to creditors and increasing the amount the business owes its owners.

The categories and format of the balance sheet are established by a system known as generally accepted accounting principles (GAAP). The system is applied to all companies, large or small, so anyone reading the balance sheet can readily understand the story it tells.

Assets

An asset is anything the business owns that has monetary value. Fixed assets are assets of the business that will retain value over a number of years. These include tangible assets such as freehold property, leasehold property, equipment, fixtures and fittings, improvements made to the property, and motor vehicles. Also included within fixed assets are "intangible" assets such as goodwill (the value of the name and reputation of the business, normally acquired when purchasing an established practice). Within most financial statements there will be a separate schedule prepared in respect of the fixed assets of the business.

A typical fixed asset schedule shows:
• The historic cost of each individual asset.
• The accumulated depreciation (i.e. deterioration in value in respect of each asset at the commencement of that particular trading period).
• Detail in terms of the further depreciation charged in that particular trading year.

It can therefore be seen that the difference between the original cost and the accumulated depreciation is the written-down value of each asset.

Current assets include not only cash, stocks of materials and saleable goods, but also money due from patients, the Dental Practice Board or other businesses (known as accounts receivable or debtors) and prepaid expenses relating to the next financial period.

Liabilities

Liabilities are monies owed by the business. These are often split into current and long-term liabilities. Current liabilities can be money the business owes either for products purchased or services received but not paid for at the time of receipt of these goods (creditors). Liabilities can also be negative bank balances, credit card balances and monies owed on hire purchase agreements due within one year. Long-term liabilities are liabilities that have a maturity date of greater than one year. These typically include bank loans, mortgages, hire purchase agreements and any other liabilities maturing in greater than one year.

The owner's equity (or net worth or capital) is the money put into a business by its owners for use by the business in acquiring assets, less any money taken out of the business (drawings). At any given time, a business's assets equal the total contributions by the creditors and owners, as illustrated by the following formula for the balance sheet:

$$\text{assets} = \text{liabilities} + \text{net worth}.$$

This formula is a basic premise of accounting. If a business owes more money to creditors than it possesses in value of assets owned, the net worth or owner's equity of the business will be a negative figure.

Net Worth

Net worth is the assets of the business minus its liabilities. Net worth equals the owner's equity. This equity is the investment by the owner, plus any profits or minus any losses that have accumulated in the business

The Profit-and-Loss Account

This is also known as the income and expenditure account. It can be looked upon as a sort of financial history book, which gives a summarised form of the result of the year's trading. On newly developing practices it is especially useful to prepare profit-and-loss accounts as often as possible. This will allow problems to be identified early, thereby allowing timely intervention to avoid the problem escalating. Quarterly or even monthly management accounts are often prepared by the better-managed practices.

The profit-and-loss account can be used to identify problem areas and trends within the practice. This is achieved by comparing the profit and loss to previous periods and calculating margins and ratios. Accountants experienced in the business of dentistry should be able to advice on what margins and ratios the practice should be achieving.

Another useful exercise, especially on a newly developed practice where previous periods are not available for comparison, is benchmarking the accounts of the practice to other practices. This involves comparing the key performance ratios of the practice to those of other similar practices. By analysing the differences in the ratios achieved it is possible to identify areas where the practice is underachieving or overspending. Your accountant should be able to advise you on this.

Financial Ratios and Benchmarking

Any assessment of a practice's performance is likely to include a look at the practice's performance in previous years, and a comparison with other practices (benchmarking). The use of percentages and of various ratios helps in the assessment of trends and in comparison with other practices, and in particular may highlight aspects of a practice that merit closer scrutiny.

There are four basic ways in which one item of financial information can be related to another:

- A line-by-line comparison can be made of the current year's accounts with those of the previous year.
- The above analysis can be extended over several years (usually limited to five).
- Balance-sheet items can be expressed as a percentage of the balance sheet total and each profit-and-loss account item as a percentage of fees earned (sometimes called vertical analysis).
- Comparing one item in a balance sheet or profit and loss account with another for the same period can produce ratios.

Comparison with the previous year
This is possibly the simplest method of comparing one year's figures with another and involves working out the percentage change from the previous year of each main component of the accounts. Percentage changes in themselves may reveal a certain amount about a practice's performance but they are of most value in prompting further enquiry.

Comparison over several years
A summary of, say, the last five year's accounts can be very useful for a quick analysis of trends, even if a more detailed look is subsequently needed (see Appendix 2). Figs 8-1, 8-2 and 8-3 show graphs that have been created using standard spreadsheet software with the information contained in Appendix 2 to show year-on-year trends.

The main drawback to any analysis of trends over several years in times of high inflation is that the figures can be very misleading, with static or even declining performance in real terms (having removed the effects of inflation) appearing to have an upward trend in the figures. Comparing the trend of fees earned and profit with the trend in the retail price index can give a rough idea of the effects of inflation over the years.

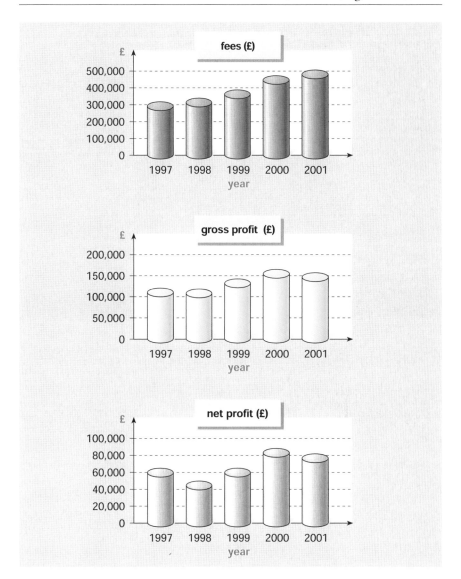

Fig 8-1 Graphs illustrating fees, gross profit and net profit.

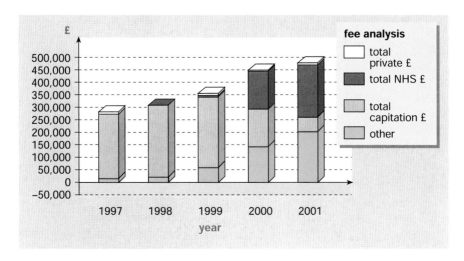

Fig 8-2 Graph illustrating fee analysis.

One last point to note is that if the rate of growth is fast, which it may be in the early years of the life of a practice, the figures year by year can give the impression that the practice's growth is accelerating when it may in fact be slowing down, when expressed as a year-on-year percentage. This is shown in Table 8-1.

Vertical analysis
The advantages of vertical analysis are that items are reduced to a common scale for inter-practice comparisons and changes in structure of a practice stand out more clearly. For example, the direct costs of a practice may remain

Table 8-1. **Rate of growth expressed as a year-on-year percentage**

Year	1998	1999	2000	2001	2002
Profit	£100,000	£130,000	£166,000	£206,000	£248,000
Year's increase		£30,000	£36,000	£40,000	£42,000
Percentage increase over previous year		30%	27.7%	24.1%	20.4%

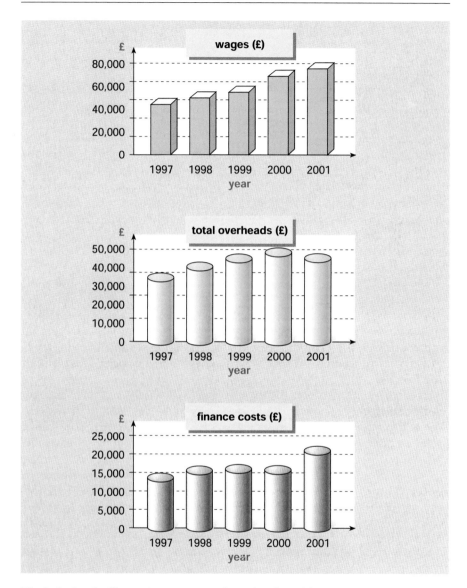

Fig 8-3 Graphs illustrating wages, total overheads and finance costs.

static over, say, five years but the constituent parts of a practice's total direct costs may change significantly over the same period.

The use of ratios

With both a balance sheet and a profit-and-loss account each containing a minimum of ten to twenty items, the scope for comparing one item with another is enormous. It is important to be selective, both to limit the calculations required and, more importantly, to make the presentation of the selected ratios simple and easily understood. No decision-maker wants a jungle of figures, so the ratios chosen should be the key ones, logically grouped.

Ratios can be conveniently divided into two main groups: operating ratios and financial ratios. Operating ratios are concerned with how the practice is trading, and take no account of how the practice is financed. Financial ratios measure the financial structure of the practice and show how it relates to trading activities.

Financial Ratios

The main operating ratios are:
- trading profit/fees = profit margin, expressed as a percentage
- gross profit/fees = gross profit margin, expressed as a percentage.

Direct costs, such as materials, lab fees, payroll, associates' fees, hygienists' fees can be expressed as a ratio of total fee income. By dividing the expenditure on each item by the gross fee income, you can express your direct costs as a percentage of gross fee income (see Appendix 3).

Financial ratios fall into two broad groups: gearing and liquidity. Gearing is concerned with the proportion of capital employed in a practice that is borrowed while liquidity ratios are concerned with a practice's cash position. A practice with "low gearing" is one financed predominantly by money introduced by the owner, whereas a "highly geared" practice is one that relies heavily on borrowings for a significant proportion of its capital. The trading profit of a practice that is highly geared is more sensitive to changes in interest rates than a lower-geared practice.

The ratio most commonly used in assessing a practice's liquidity is concerned with current assets (stocks, work-in-progress, debtors and cash) and current liabilities (creditors, bank overdraft and any debts due to be settled within the next twelve months). A practice's current ratio is current assets/current liabilities and is a broad indicator of a company's short-term financial position: a ratio of more than 1 indicates a surplus of current assets over current liabilities. A current ratio of about 1.5 is regarded as prudent in order to maintain creditworthiness. A higher figure is not necessarily a good sign – it may indicate excessive stocks or debtors or that the owner is sitting on an unduly large amount of cash, which could be more profitably invested.

The most informative feature of a current ratio is its normal level and any trend from year to year. A drop below normal levels is worth investigating, and a continuing decline is a warning signal that should not be ignored.

Benchmarking

As well as assessing a practice's own performance, ratios can also be used to compare performance with other, similar practices. For years, organisations have been using benchmarking to see how they compare with the best in their industry, not only in financial terms but also in areas such as management and marketing. By benchmarking a dental practice with practices having a similar structure and fee mix it is possible to highlight areas that should be investigated further and addressed if the practice is to achieve its full potential. Benchmarking is only a means to an end – being made aware of performance gaps is of considerable value in itself, but it is acting upon the findings where the real benefit lies. As with ratio analysis, benchmarking is not a one-off process. To be effective, it must be done on a regular basis.

Chapter 9
Investment and Protections

However successful you are in the business of dentistry, it is always important to keep your financial circumstances and requirements under review at all times. There is no doubt that too few practitioners review their financial position often enough.

There are many various forms of insurance, which are available to protect you and your family in terms of replacing income and paying off debts in the event of misfortune. Protection plans such as permanent health insurance, critical illness cover and life assurance should all be used to protect you, your assets and your family. A detailed analysis of protection plans and investment strategy is beyond the scope of the present text, but there are many specialist advisers who will be able to assist you with your requirements.

Permanent Health Insurance

Permanent health insurance provides for a replacement income in the event of injury or disability. Insurance companies will allow you to insure a percentage of your income, normally up to a maximum of around 70% (this varies from company to company). The benefits of the plan can also be deferred so that they begin either on day one, or after four, 13, 26 or 52 weeks.

Practice Overheads Plan

This type of arrangement is renewable each year, and provides an income to ensure that the practice can continue to run in the event of you being absent from the practice due to sickness or accident.

Critical Illness Cover

The development of critical illness insurance has been a major breakthrough in terms of providing enhanced protection to individuals and their dependants. In financial terms, the onset of a critical illness can be even more traumatic than death and therefore your individual cover and protection must be reviewed routinely. Critical illness cover provides a lump sum payment on the diagnosis of any one of a range of illnesses specified in the policy when taken out. A general list of illnesses covered is given here, although this may vary from policy to policy:

- heart attack
- kidney failure
- cancer
- stroke
- permanent total disability.

Most insurers will also pay out if treatment is required under the following circumstances:

- coronary artery bypass
- major organ transplant.

Critical illness cover is normally written in conjunction with life cover protection (see below) and it is now accepted that most practitioners require cover for critical illness as well as significant life assurance cover to protect their practice investment and financial liabilities, as well as their dependants.

Life Assurance

The cheapest form of life assurance is term cover and this is a simple and relatively cheap way to make sure that any liabilities you may have are covered in the event of your death. A life assurance plan will provide a lump sum payment on your death in return for a regular payment to an insurance company. This type of plan is used to cover your mortgage, practice purchase and any other liabilities such as loans for practice equipment purchase or even a car loan.

Apart from basic life and critical illness cover there are alternative forms of life assurance, which allow for an element of investment. Such policies are either with-profit endowments or unit-linked assurance to provide a minimum level of death benefit, together with a growing investment fund that is normally payable upon maturity. The returns on such investments are not guaranteed and it is therefore important to understand that such policies work best over relatively long periods of time.

There is also "whole of life" cover that guarantees a certain amount of benefit payable upon death and can be written on an individual as well as a joint-life basis. Such policies are particularly useful in terms of providing funds to beneficiaries for the payment of inheritance tax (see below).

Retirement Planning

Once the policies are in place to cover you in the event of illness or death, the next stage is to ensure that you can retire when you want and at the level of income that you require. It cannot be over-stressed that the earlier you start planning for retirement the better, and if you delay planning even by a year, this can have a significant impact upon your retirement plans. If you intend to retire early with a significant income in retirement then very substantial investment is required as soon as funds permit.

Pension planning has become more difficult recently because of the fact that most pension funds are growing at a lower rate than was previously the case. That said, we are enjoying a period of relatively low inflation and therefore the investment growth requirement is not as high now as it used to be. Investment in pensions at the right level throughout your working life should ensure that you have your desired income in retirement. However, this needs constant review and alteration to make sure that your continued investment is at the correct level.

It is particularly important to be fully aware of the benefits of the NHS superannuation scheme and how contributions to the NHS scheme can impact on your ability to contribute to retirement annuity or personal pension plans. Advice must therefore be obtained from those financial advisors who fully understand this complicated area.

Group Personal Pension Plan or Stakeholder Pension Scheme

Whilst you are not obliged to make payments to a group personal pension plan or stakeholder pension scheme, establishing a scheme and contributing to it can provide a worthwhile reward for any staff you employ and will help to promote loyalty to the business. Administering a staff pension scheme can be a complex and time-consuming affair, so a group personal pension plan or stakeholder scheme may give you the flexibility that you require and demand less employer administration that any of the available alternatives.

Executive Pension Plan

This type of plan is taken out by the employer for a key employee, to fund a pension scheme for them based on these earnings. There are certain tax benefits on this type of pension scheme. However, the scheme can be complex and the pension fund belongs to the pension trustees as opposed to the employee. At retirement, an income is purchased by the pension trustees for the employee.

Savings and Investments

There are various vehicles available for savings and investments. These range from National Savings products to Friendly Society plans to insurance company bonds and regular savings plans. You can also utilise individual savings accounts (ISAs), which can be used to provide either tax-free income or tax-free growth or a mixture of the two.

If you wish to invest on a regular basis or have a lump sum to invest, it is important to ensure that your investment is structured in the correct way. This should take account of your attitude to risk and any tax advantages that are available.

Partnership Assurance

The purpose of employing this type of policy is to provide sufficient funds for you or your business partner(s) to purchase your (or their) interest in the business from your (or their) estate in the event of the death of one of you. In order to ensure that the policy proceeds are paid into the right hands at the right time and used for the correct purpose, the beneficiaries should be your partner(s), provided that you and they are both still involved in the business at that time. It is advisable to take legal advice to ensure that the plans are set up correctly, so that there are no problems in the event of a claim being made.

Inheritance Tax

Once the correct level of protection and the requirements of your retirement have been established, focus is then required on the value of your estate and the tax-efficient transfer of this to your relatives. The situation in respect of married couples is very straightforward as most wills pass on the value of the deceased's estate to the surviving spouse and there is no liability to inheritance tax on such transfers. The real problem starts when the surviving spouse dies and it is at that point that Inland Revenue can become very interested in the value of the second estate.

The recent growth in the value of residential property has created a greater problem for many taxpayers and although there has been pressure on the Government to exempt certain elements of domestic property from the inheritance tax calculation, recent Budgets have not delivered at all in this regard. It therefore remains the case that once an estate exceeds £250,000 the excess above this figure can be subject to tax at 40%. There are certain reliefs to mitigate some of the tax charge but the fact remains that most estates are fully chargeable above the threshold figure.

For example:

value of the estate	£1,000,000
nil rate band	£ 250,000
taxable estate	£ 750,000

Assuming that the estate is fully chargeable, the tax payable would be £300,000, leaving a net estate of £700,000 to the beneficiaries of the deceased. The effective tax charge on this case is still 30% of the total value of the estate. (The above calculation assumes tax rates and exemptions applying from 6 April 2002 and are subject to change in future Budgets.)

Sensible planning can substantially reduce, and often eradicate, the charge to tax, thus leaving substantially more to the relatives than would otherwise have been the case. Such planning can extend to putting assets and insurance policies in trust for your relatives, removing them from the value of the estate for the purposes of inheritance tax, achieving tax-free transfer of the value.

As with all financial matters, careful planning and professional advice are essential at all times. Advice should therefore be sought from an independent financial advisor (IFA). It is now becoming increasingly common that such advice is provided on a fee basis with all initial commissions either being rebated or reinvested for the benefit of the investor. Reinvestment of commission can make a significant difference to fund growth, particularly in terms of pension investment.

It must, therefore, be understood that the sensible practice owner will review their protections and investments on an annual basis. Individual circumstances do change significantly over time and it is only by assessing the individual protection requirements and the funds available for investment that sensible financial planning can be achieved.

Personal Accident Insurance

There are other insurances that you may not have realised can provide you with additional protection, albeit for your family and practice. As a dentist, the thought of an accident that could result in the loss of the use of a hand or the sight of an eye is not something that you want to dwell on. It is even more of a concern if such an accident prevents you from continuing with your chosen career. Personal accident insurance will provide a substantial lump sum benefit in the event of such a disability. This lump sum will allow you clear any outstanding business loans and may even help in training for a new career.

Appendix 1 Financial statements

DR JOE BLOGGS

FINANCIAL STATEMENTS

FOR YEAR ENDED 30 APRIL 2003

DR JOE BLOGGS

GENERAL INFORMATION
FOR YEAR ENDED 30 APRIL 2003

PROPRIETOR   Dr Joe Bloggs

ADDRESS   1 The Street
London W1

ACCOUNTANTS   Dental Business Solutions
Network House
Station Yard
THAME
Oxon OX9 3UH

DR JOE BLOGGS

TRADING AND PROFIT AND LOSS ACCOUNT
FOR YEAR ENDED 30 APRIL 2003

	2003		2002	
	£	£	£	£
Fees		**472,493**		444,270
Direct costs				
Opening Stock	**4,286**		4,201	
Dental Materials	**58,110**		45,803	
Laboratory Fees	**33,902**		30,807	
Associate Fees	**133,237**		129,346	
Hygienist Fees	**24,256**		10,540	
Wages	**74,876**		67,756	
	328,667		288,453	
Closing Stock	**(5,390)**		(4,286)	
		323,277		284,167
GROSS PROFIT		**149,216**		160,103
Other income				
Interest Received		**169**		149
		149,385		160,252
Overheads				
Telephone	**1,910**		1,444	
Postage & Stationery	**5,461**		5,626	
Motor Expenses	**3,285**		2,367	
Subscriptions & Courses	**1,457**		2,610	
Computer Expenses	**2,678**		1,749	

Equipment Maintenance	**1,708**		1,370
Cleaning Laundry & Uniforms	**7,222**		7,566
Sundry Expenses	**3,592**		2,136
Accountancy & Professional	**4,998**		7,498
Advertising	**1,057**		1,426
Superannuation	**186**		1,178
Rates	**1,973**		1,662
Use of Home as Office	**642**		642
Insurance	**2,475**		2,195
Light & Heat	**1,536**		1,422
Repairs & Renewals	**4,285**		6,512
		44,465	47,403
		104,920	112,849

Finance costs

Loan Interest	**9,057**		9,118
Hire Purchase Interest	**1,214**		1,255
Rental of Equipment	**7,638**		1,672
Bank Charges	**2,487**		3,175
		20,396	15,220
Carried forward		**84,524**	97,629

DR JOE BLOGGS

TRADING AND PROFIT AND LOSS ACCOUNT
FOR YEAR ENDED 30 APRIL 2003

	2003		2002	
	£	£	£	£
Brought forward		**84,524**		97,629
Depreciation				
Equip Fixtures & Fittings	**5,043**		4,218	
Motor Vehicles	**2,039**		2,039	
Computer Equipment	**2,186**		8,181	
		9,268		14,438
		75,256		83,191
Profit on disposal of fixed assets				
Disposal of Assets		**200**		36
NET PROFIT		**£75,456**		£83,227

DR JOE BLOGGS

BALANCE SHEET
30 APRIL 2003

	2003			2002
	£	**£**	£	£
FIXED ASSETS				
Goodwill	**66,500**		66,500	
Freehold Property	**62,500**		62,500	
Improvements to Property	**13,207**		11,706	
Equipment Fixtures & Fittings	**13,019**		8,645	
Motor Vehicles	**6,117**		8,156	
Computer Equipment	**1,791**		3,065	
		163,134		160,572
CURRENT ASSETS				
Stock	**5,390**		4,286	
Trade Debtors	**9,287**		10,347	
Prepayments & Accrued Income	**106**		106	
Current Bank Account	**6,716**		3,346	
Reserve Capital Account	**3,006**		–	
Business High Interest Account	**343**		9,786	
Cash in Hand	**115**		115	
	24,963		27,986	
CURRENT LIABILITIES				
Trade Creditors	**29,347**		25,147	
Hire Purchase Creditor	**5,494**		9,173	
	34,841		34,320	
		(9,878)		(6,334)
		£153,256		£154,238

FINANCED BY

LONG TERM LIABILITIES

Bank Loans			**97,565**		108,728

CAPITAL ACCOUNT

Balance brought forward	**45,510**			36,766	
Add					
Net profit	**75,456**			83,227	
	120,966			119,993	
Less					
Drawings	**65,275**			74,483	
		55,691			45,510
		£153,256			£154,238

DR JOE BLOGGS

INTANGIBLE FIXED ASSETS SCHEDULE
30 APRIL 2003

	Goodwill
	£
COST	
At 1 May 2002	
and 30 April 2003	**66,500**
NET BOOK VALUE	
At 30 April 2003	**66,500**
At 30 April 2002	**66,500**

DR JOE BLOGGS

TANGIBLE FIXED ASSETS SCHEDULE
30 APRIL 2003

	Freehold Property	Improvements to Property	Equipment Fixtures & Fittings
	£	£	£
COST			
At 1 May 2002	62,500	11,706	43,460
Additions	-	1,501	9,417
At 30 April 2003	62,500	13,207	52,877
DEPRECIATION			
At 1 May 2002	-	-	34,815
Charge for year	-	-	5,043
At 30 April 2003	-	-	39,858
NET BOOK VALUE			
At 30 April 2003	62,500	13,207	13,019
At 30 April 2002	62,500	11,706	8,645

	Motor Vehicles	Computer Equipment	Totals
	£	£	£
COST			
At 1 May 2002	10,195	24,543	152,404
Additions	-	911	11,829
At 30 April 2003	10,195	25,454	164,233

DEPRECIATION

At 1 May 2002	**2,039**	**21,477**	**58,331**
Charge for year	**2,039**	**2,186**	**9,268**
At 30 April 2003	**4,078**	**23,663**	**67,599**

NET BOOK VALUE

At 30 April 2003	**6,117**	**1,791**	**96,634**
At 30 April 2002	8,156	3,065	94,072

Appendix 2 Five –year financial summary

DR JOE BLOGGS

5 YEAR FINANCIAL SUMMARY

PRINCIPAL

30 APRIL 2003

Year	5	4	3	2	1
Profit & Loss					
Fees	472,493	444,270	353,156	304,127	279,441
Cost of Sales					
Dental Materials	57,006	45,718	29,191	26,526	24,215
Laboratory Fees	33,902	30,807	29,191	26,526	24,215
Associate Fees	133,237	129,346	101,073	87,361	66,498
Hygienest Fees	24,256	10,540	3,777	3,845	3,898
Wages	74,876	67,756	54,564	50,561	43,494
Locum Fees & Others			981		
Total Cost of Sales	323,277	284,167	219,570	194,859	166,208
Gross Profit	149,216	160,103	133,586	109,268	113,233
Other Income	169	149	134	1,278	123
Total Overheads	44,465	47,403	44,691	39,633	34,906
Operating Profit	104,920	112,849	89,029	70,913	78,450
Finance Costs	20,396	15,220	15,552	15,333	13,144
Depreciation	9,068	14,402	13,279	12,460	5,630
Net Profit	75,456	83,227	60,198	43,120	59,676
Balance Sheet					
Intangible fixed assets	66,500	66,500	66,500	66,500	66,500
Tangible fixed assets	96,634	94,072	83,382	93,355	79,439
Total fixed assets	163,134	160,572	149,882	159,855	145,939
Stock	5,390	4,286	4,201		
Trade debtors	9,287	10,347	18,277	19,145	21,486
Cash & bank balances	10,180	13,247	17,313	7,765	6,794
Other Assets	106	106	1,288	235	14,281
Current Assets	24,963	27,986	41,079	27,145	42,561
Trade creditors	29,347	25,147	22,577	12,684	14,338
Borrowings – Within 1 year					
Other Liabilities – Within 1 year	5,494	9,173	16,183	15,733	999
Current Liabilities	34,841	34,320	38,760	28,417	15,337
Borrowings – Greater than 1 year	97,565	108,728	115,437	125,087	134,654
Total Liabilities after 1 year	97,565	108,728	115,437	125,087	134,654

| **Total Liabilities** | 132,406 | 143,048 | 154,197 | 153,504 | 149,991 |
| **Net Assets** | 55,691 | 45,510 | 36,764 | 33,496 | 38,509 |

Capital Account

| Opening balance | 45,510 | 36,766 | 33,496 | 38,506 | 44,398 |
| Net Profit | 75,456 | 83,227 | 60,198 | 43,120 | 59,676 |

| Capital Introduced | | | | | |
| Less Drawings | 65,275 | 74,483 | 56,930 | 48,133 | 65,565 |

Appendix 3 Cost expressed as percentage of fees

DR JOE BLOGGS

TABLE OF RESULTS

PRINCIPAL

30 APRIL 2003

Year	5	4	3	2	1
Gross Fees	£472,493	£444,270	£353,156	£304,127	£279,441
Gross Profit(%)	32	36	38	36	41
Cost as percentage of fees					
Wages	16	15	15	17	16
Materials	12	10	8	9	9
Laboratary Fees	7	7	8	9	10
Associate/Locum fees	28	29	29	29	24
Hygienist fees	5	2	1	1	1
Overhead costs	9	11	13	13	12
Finance costs	4	3	4	5	5
Depreciation	2	3	4	4	2
Net profit (%)	16	19	17	14	21
Net profit	£75,456	£83,227	£60,198	£43,120	£59,676
Drawings	£65,275	£74,483	£56,930	£48,133	£65,565
other income	£169	£149	£134	£1,2789	£123

Index

Quintessentials for General Dental Practitioners Series

in 36 volumes

Editor-in-Chief: Professor Nairn H F Wilson

The Quintessentials for General Dental Practitioners Series covers basic principles and key issues in all aspects of modern dental medicine. Each book can be read as a stand-alone volume or in conjunction with other books in the series.

Publication date,
approximately

Oral Surgery and Oral Medicine, Editor: John G Meechan

Practical Dental Local Anaesthesia	available
Practical Oral Medicine	Spring 2004
Practical Conscious Sedation	Autumn 2003
Practical Surgical Dentistry	Spring 2004

Imaging, Editor: Keith Horner

Interpreting Dental Radiographs	available
Panoramic Radiology	Autumn 2003
Twenty-first Century Dental Imaging	Autumn 2004

Periodontology, Editor: Iain L C Chapple

Understanding Periodontal Diseases: Assessment and Diagnostic Procedures in Practice	available
Decision-Making for the Periodontal Team	Autumn 2003
Successful Periodontal Therapy – A Non-Surgical Approach	Autumn 2003
Periodontal Management of Children and Adolescents	Autumn 2003
Periodontal Medicine in Practice	Spring 2004

Implantology, Editor: Lloyd J Searson

Implants for the General Practitioner	available
Managing Orofacial Pain in General Dental Practice	Spring 2003

Endodontics, Editor: John M Whitworth

Rational Root Canal Treatment in Practice	available
Managing Endodontic Failure in Practice	Autumn 2003
Managing Dental Trauma in Practice	Autumn 2003
Managing the Vital Pulp in Practice	Autumn 2004

Prosthodontics, Editor: P Finbarr Allen

Teeth for Life for Older Adults	available
Complete Dentures – from Planning to Problem Solving	Autumn 2003
Removable Partial Dentures – A Systematic Approach	Autumn 2003
Fixed Prosthodontics for the General Dental Practitioner	Autumn 2003
Occlusion: A Theoretical and Team Approach	Autumn 2004

Operative Dentistry, Editor: Paul A Brunton

Decision-Making in Operative Dentistry	available
Applied Dental Materials in Operative Dentistry	Spring 2003
Aesthetic Dentistry	Autumn 2003
Successful Indirect Restorations in General Practice	Spring 2004

Paediatric Dentistry/Orthodontics, Editor: Marie Therese Hosey

Child Taming: How to Cope with Children in Dental Practice	Spring 2003
Paediatric Cariology	Autumn 2003
Treatment Planning for the Developing Dentition	Autumn 2003

General Dentistry and Practice Management, Editor: Raj Rattan

The Business of Dentistry	available
Risk Management in General Dental Practice	Spring 2003
Practice Management for the Dental Team	Autumn 2003
Application of Information Technology in General Dental Practice	Spring 2004
Quality Assurance in General Dental Practice	Autumn 2004
Evidence-Based Care in General Dental Practice	Spring 2005

Quintessence Publishing Co. Ltd., London